Diabetic
Eye Disease

Previously published as *Don't Go Blind from Diabetes*

Diabetic Eye Disease

An easy to understand guide to keeping
your vision for people with diabetes

David Khorram, MD

Director Emeritus, Center for Diabetic Eye Care

Marianas Eye Institute

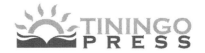

Cover design by Maria Carla Alegria (2013), updated by Jordan Raj (2018)

Book design by Velin Saramov

ISBN-13: 978-0-9800531-2-8
ISBN-10: 0-9800531-2-9

Published by Tiningo Press

Printed in the United States of America

Dedicated to the peoples of the Mariana Islands, who have graciously allowed me the privilege of serving them and being a part of their lives.

And to my parents, my father, Dr. Houshang Khorram, whose gentle passion for serving his patients inspired me to become a doctor. I have always hoped to practice my profession by the example he set before me – with warmth, compassion, humor and true joy. And to my mother, Tabendeh "Toby" Khorram, whose dedication to her faith, and whose patience and perseverance in sharing knowledge to improve her community, have served as a guiding example for me.

ACKNOWLEDGEMENTS

This second edition is made possible through the diligent work of Alice Sicong Liu. I met Alice in Africa during the summer of 2016. At the time she was a promising undergraduate student entering her third year at Duke University. We were both part of a volunteer project to combat blindness in rural Ghana. Alice had already been in Ghana for two months when I arrived. I was immediately struck by her generous and devoted spirit, her calm and positive attitude in often trying circumstances, her sense of adventure and curiosity, her warmth for the peoples and cultures around her, and her keen intellect. I knew immediately that I wanted to continue to collaborate with Alice, so I invited her to undertake revising this book. I am grateful that she accepted. She contributed improvements to the entire book, and her significant contributions to chapters 3 and 20 merit that she be listed as a co-author of those chapters. Thank you, Alice.

Contents

INTRODUCTION

In over twenty years of taking care of thousands of people with diabetic eye disease, I have seen many of these people tragically go blind. Diabetes in rare cases is relentless and difficult to combat. But in most of my patients, they didn't have to lose vision. They lost their vision not purely because they had diabetes, but because they didn't understand the disease. They didn't know the importance of an eye exam, or they waited for symptoms to appear before they came to see me, or they didn't come back for follow up care, or they were too scared to get the treatment they needed. Through all this, I have found that the more you know about diabetic eye disease, the more likely you are to get the care you need, and to keep your vision.

I tried to find a book about diabetic eye disease that I could give my patients, so they would gain the knowledge they needed. The books that I found were either outdated, or far too technical. I was surprised that nothing existed that was up-to-date, complete, and easy to understand. So, I decided to write this book. I wrote it for my patients, and I wrote it for you – to give you the knowledge you need to protect your vision from diabetes, to calm your fears and anxieties, to give you peace of mind and hope, to give you the tools you need to understand your doctor, and to empower you to ask questions and participate wisely in decisions about your care.

Many people have shared with me that the book has been incredibly helpful. Since publishing the first edition, new research results and new technologies have become available, and so, it is time for this revised and updated edition.

This book contains a lot of important information, but if you don't remember anything else, I ask you to take three fairly simple actions that can save your vision. First, get an eye exam, even if your vision seems okay. Second, keep your follow-up appointments. And, third, get the treatment that your doctor recommends. If you take these three actions, you'll be well on your way to keeping your vision for a lifetime.

I've written this book in the same every-day language that I use when I talk with patients. You will know most of the words, but when a medical word is used for the first time, it is *italicized* and explained. I expect that you may skip around as you read this book. For this reason, I repeat some of the basic concepts and definitions from chapter to chapter. As an additional help, the glossary at the end of the book contains common words and abbreviations used when talking about diabetic eye disease.

The first part of this book explains how diabetes causes damage throughout the body, with special attention to the eye. I show you how the eye works. I discuss the major form of diabetic eye disease, *diabetic retinopathy*. I also explain other common eye diseases associated with diabetes, such as cataracts, fluctuating vision, and double vision.

In part two, I explain each step of the eye exam – how to prepare for a visit to the eye doctor, the major parts of the exam, specials tests you may need, and the critical importance of your follow-up visits.

Part three reviews treatments available and what you can expect from each. The last few years have opened an exciting era in the treatment of diabetic retinopathy. New drug discoveries have given us powerful tools to save your vision and to reverse some of the vision loss caused by diabetes.

In the last part of the book, I share with you the importance of controlling diabetes, and its companion diseases: obesity, high blood pressure, high cholesterol, and smoking. Addressing these diseases is key to preventing blindness. Although it is beyond the scope of this book to delve into all of these issues in detail, I hope this brief introduction encourages you to learn more.

Use this book as a companion. Come back to it as often as you like. I know that your time with your doctor can be limited. If you're anything like me, even when the doctor explains things completely, the minute you leave the doctor's office, you forget half of what was said, and remember twice as many questions that you meant to ask. I will be here, to explain things again.

I spend a lot of my time explaining the complexities of diabetic eye disease to my patients. "Thank you Doctor, now I understand," are among the sweetest words I hear. I hope that you find my explanations as clear as my patients do. I have done my best to take the most important information – the stuff you need to know in order to keep your vision – and share it with you in a clear and easy to understand way. Now, come, and let's start a journey that will give you the knowledge you need so you don't go blind from diabetes and so you keep your vision for life.

ABOUT
THE AUTHOR

D avid Khorram, MD, is a board-certified ophthalmolo-gist, educator, speaker, and writer. After completing his training at Northwestern University in Chicago, he spent over twenty years in the South Pacific developing eye care in the Mariana Islands. There, on the island of Saipan, he established the Center for Diabetic Eye Care at Marianas Eye Institute, and participated in the Diabetic Retinopathy Clinical Research Network. He has published scientific arti-cles in the peer-reviewed journals, *Ophthalmology, Archives of Ophthalmology, American Journal of Ophthalmology, Ophthalmic Surgery and Lasers,* and *Molecular Vision.* He is listed in *Guide to America's Top Ophthalmologists.*

Dr. Khorram is also the co-founders of Brilliant Star Mon-tessori School, a non-profit school on Saipan. He is the au-thor of the award-winning book, *World Peace, a Blind Wife, and Gecko Tails,* which has been used for many years as required reading in sociology classes at the University of Guam. Dr.

Khorram's interests lie in global healthcare and capacity-building. He serves as a volunteer surgeon and instructor for eye care projects and programs around the world.

PART I

DIABETES AND THE EYE

In this section you will learn the effects of diabetes on the eye. In the first chapter you'll learn about diabetes, and how it damages organs throughout your body. The damage is related to high blood sugar, or what is also called high blood *glucose*. Throughout the book, sometimes I'll say "sugar" and sometimes, "glucose." They mean the same thing.

The second chapter will give you a general understanding of the way the eye works, and what happens to a beam of light as it passes into your eye.

Next, you'll learn about the amazing retina, that delicate structure that coats the inside of the eye and is at particular risk of damage from diabetes.

After this, I'll take you on a tour of diabetic retinopathy, describing the damage that diabetes causes to the retina. There are three separate chapters discussing diabetic retinopathy: one on the early stages of diabetic retinopathy, one on macular edema, and one on proliferative diabetic retinopathy. (You'll learn what all these words mean in the chapters to come.)

Usually when we doctors talk about diabetic eye disease, we're talking about diabetic retinopathy. But diabetes can affect the eye in other ways as well. I'll close this section by explaining several other eye problems that can be related to diabetes: cataracts, fluctuating vision, and double vision.

I hope that as you read these chapters, you will understand that a lot of the damage from diabetes can happen without you knowing about it. Right now, as you're reading this, damage may be taking place inside your eyes. Getting an eye exam is the first step you can take to help protect your vision.

1

How Does Diabetes Cause Damage?

You probably know that diabetes is a disease characterized by high blood sugar. It's the high blood sugar that causes damage throughout your body. But how? Your body is made up of cells that combine to form tissues, which in turn combine to form organs. The cells of your body need oxygen to stay alive and to do their job.

Blood Vessels Carry Oxygen

When you take a breath, your lungs take in the air around you and extract the oxygen from it. Your lungs then transfer the oxygen to your blood. Your heart pumps this oxygen-rich blood all through your body. The blood travels from the heart to the cells through a system of blood vessels. The blood vessels that emerge from the heart are very large, and as they move farther from the heart, they branch many times, to become smaller and smaller, much like the branches of a tree.

The tiniest blood vessels are called *capillaries*. The capillaries are like the twigs feeding the leaves. They carry the oxygen-rich blood to the cells and tissues awaiting the oxygen.

Diabetes Damages Blood Vessels

Without oxygen, the cells can't work properly; the tissues sustain damage and the organs that are made up of those cells die. High blood sugar damages blood vessels. We don't understand exactly how the damage occurs, but we do know that when the blood vessels are damaged, oxygen cannot be delivered efficiently to the cells and they die. Most damage from diabetes happens through this process – high blood sugar causes damage to blood vessels which results in poor blood flow, blockage of blood vessels, and poor oxygen delivery to cells and tissues, which in turn leads to their dysfunction or death.

For example, the high blood sugar from diabetes damages the small blood vessels in the feet, leading to amputations. High blood sugar damages the small blood vessels in the kidneys, causing kidney failure, leading to the need for dialysis. High blood sugar damages the small blood vessels in the heart and the brain, causing heart attacks and strokes. And high blood sugar damages the small blood vessels in the eyes, causing vision loss and blindness. The complications from diabetes are caused by high blood sugar and its resulting damage to small blood vessels through the body. The damaged blood vessels cannot deliver the oxygen, and the cells die. When the cells die, the tissues and organs can't work properly. This is why controlling blood sugar is so important.

2

How Does the Eye Work?

The human eye is not only one of the most beautiful organs in the body, but also one of the most amazing structures in the universe. In this tiny space – your eye – millions of cells and connections work together to allow you to sense colors, shapes, movement, depth and brightness. The eyes bring the distant world to you. They bring twinkling stars, red sunsets, glimmering mountains, and the face of your loved ones from "out there," and allow you to hold them within you. I feel blessed to spend my days looking at this amazing, delicate and intricate structure. Let's take a look at how this miraculous organ works.

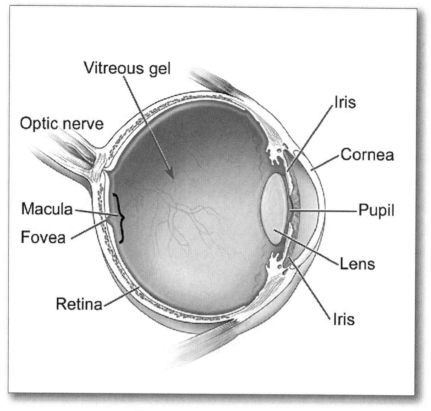

Figure 1: Parts of the eye

A Hollow Ball

I tell my patients that the eye is like a hollow ball. Light comes from outside the eye and penetrates into its deep structures where a thin layer of nerves and blood vessels turns the light into electricity, and sends the information to your brain.

Cornea and Sclera

As light reaches your eye, the first structure that it strikes is the cornea. Your cornea is the clear covering over the brown or blue part of the eye. Of all the tissues of the human body, the cornea has an exceptionally unique quality: it is perfectly clear. It allows light to pass through it. Because it's clear, it serves as a window allowing light in. Through this clear window, we can peer into the deep structures of your eye.

The cornea merges with the sclera, the white part of the eye. The sclera and the cornea together make up the wall of the eye-ball. The sclera is covered by a thin tissue called the *conjunctiva*. When your eye gets red, it is the blood vessels in the conjunctiva that are giving the red appearance.

Iris and Pupil

Right behind your cornea is the colored part of the eye, which is called the *iris*. If the iris were a solid sheet of tissue, the light could go no farther. But luckily, the iris has a hole in the middle of it. If you look in the mirror, or into someone's eye, you can see this black hole in the middle of the iris. This hole is called the *pupil*. As you watch your eye in the mirror, you may notice that the pupil changes in size. When you look at a bright light, your pupil gets smaller to limit the amount of light entering your eye. When you are in a dark environment, your pupil gets bigger, to let more light in.

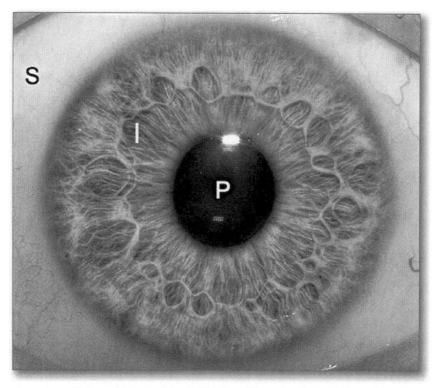

Figure 2: Photo of the front of the eye. The iris (I) is the colored tex-tured part of the eye. The center of the iris has a hole in it, the pupil (P). The iris and pupil are covered by a clear dome, the cornea. Be-cause the cornea is clear, it's not visible in the photo, but you can see a light reflection coming from the cornea, just above the "P." Right behind the pupil is the lens. The white part of the eye is the sclera (S), which is covered by a clear thin tissue called the conjunctiva. In this photo you can see a few blood vessels in the conjunctiva.

Lens

Just behind the iris is the natural *lens* of the eye. Like the cornea, the lens is clear. Light passes through it. You'll notice

24

that the cornea and the lens are both curved, and because of their curvature, they bend the rays of light as the rays pass through them. During the first half of your life, the lens is very flexible, and it can change its shape. By changing its shape, you can focus on things both far and near. But as you approach forty years old, the lens gets less flexible, and that's why you may lose the ability to see up close as you grow older. When this happens, you need reading glasses to see near objects clearly.

Vitreous

After the light passes through your cornea, pupil and lens, it passes through a large space called the *vitreous cavity* or *vitreous chamber*. This chamber is full of a jelly (called the vitreous, of course), which is usually clear, and which allows light to pass through it.

As you get older, the vitreous can form clumps, and when you see those clumps, they look like objects floating in your vision. They are called *vitreous floaters*. They are very common, and people describe them as spider webs, or bugs, or strings with beads that move around in the vision. Usually, floaters are just a natural part of getting older. But sometimes, floaters can be a sign of more severe problems, especially in people with nearsightedness or with diabetes. (If you suddenly develop floaters, or if the floaters are associated with flashing lights, see an eye specialist immediately.)

After the light passes through the vitreous, it strikes a thin layer of nerves and blood vessels that coats the inside of the eye. This layer is called the *retina*. Let's travel with a single photon of light in order to better understand the retina – a structure that is at the heart of diabetic eye disease. The retina is so important that it deserves its own chapter.

3

THE AMAZING
RETINA

Turning Light Into Electricity

Each photon of light passes though your cornea, pupil and lens, and enters the vast vitreous chamber. Like a starship traveling through space, the light heads for its target: the *retina* - that thin layer of nerves and blood vessels coating the inside of the eye. After passing through the vitreous chamber, the light crashes into your retina and penetrates its surface, heading to its deep layers. Here, below your retinal surface, the light activates the *photoreceptors* — specially designed cells that are the ultimate target of the light — which set off a chain reaction. You may have heard of these photoreceptors. There are two major kinds: the cones and the rods. Cones are responsible for your clear daytime vision and your color vision, and rods are responsible for your night vision.

The chain reactions set off by the light as it strikes your photoreceptors do an amazing thing; they change the light into an electrical signal. This newly-born electrical signal then rises back toward the surface of the retina, through a network of interconnected nerve cells. But the nerve cells don't just carry the electrical signal; they also modulate it. After all, when you look at the world, there isn't just one ray of light entering your eye at a time. Instead, wave after wave of light continuously bombard your retina. The millions of retinal cells work together, to define color, depth, shading, hue, movement, brightness and all of the other visual information flowing into your eyes. And the retinal cells do this work from second to second, as the world changes before your eyes. The most sophisticated supercomputers couldn't do the amazing work that your retina does when you simply watch someone walk by.

Turning Electricity Into Vision

As the electrical signals rise to the surface of your retina, they gather into 1.2 million nerve fibers that converge to become a small cable called the *optic nerve*. The optic nerve carries those electrical signals out of your eye and sends them toward their destination, the *occipital lobes* of your brain. Every part of the brain has different functions, and the occipital lobes, located at the back of your head, are for vision. In the occipital lobes, your brain will interpret these signals and give you the sense of sight, deciphering the millions of electrical signals into recognizable patterns — a yellow daffodil, a moving car, or your loved one's smile.

From the cornea to the brain, all the parts of your visual system must work well in order for you to see clearly. Problems with any part of the visual system can interfere with your

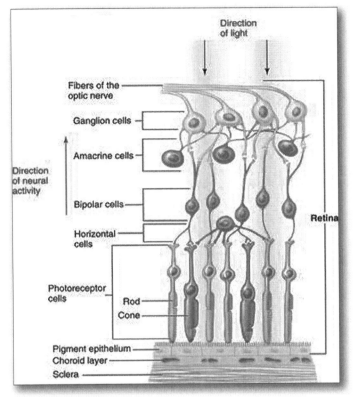

Figure 3: Layers of the retina. Light penetrates through the retinal layers to the rods and cones. The rods and cones turn light into electrical signals. The electrical signals then rise through the different nerve layers of the retina to the fibers of the optic nerve, which transmits the electrical signals to the brain. Notice that the direction of the light is toward the rods and cones, but the direction of the electrical signals (or "neural activity") is in the opposite direction.

ability to see. I often tell my patients that the eye is like an old-fashioned camera. The front parts of the eye — the cornea and the lens — focus the light. The retina is like the film inside the camera. The optic nerve delivers the film to the brain, where it is developed and turned into a picture. (For those of you more familiar with digital cameras, you can think of the retina as the CCD sensor made up of photodiodes that converts the light into electricity. The electrical signals are then sent down the optic nerve to the brain, which like the LCD screen, creates an image that you can interpret.)

What Does the Retina Look Like?

Not all regions of the retina are the same. Using an instrument called an *ophthalmoscope* (which is Latin for *thinga-ma-bob that allows us to look at the retina*) we peer through the cornea, the pupil, the lens and the vitreous chamber, and here is what we see.

Optic Disc and Blood Vessels

The brightest object in the retina is the *optic disc,* or simply, *disc.* This is the surface of the optic nerve, a collection of 1.2 million nerve fibers that leaves the eye and carries the electrical signals to your brain. Usually, the center of the optic disc is excavated and deeper than its rim. We call this excavated area of the optic disc, the *optic cup.* In the center of the disc, the major blood vessels of the retina – the arteries and veins — enter and leave your eye. On the surface of the retina we can see these blood vessels branching out, supplying oxygen to the far regions of the retina.

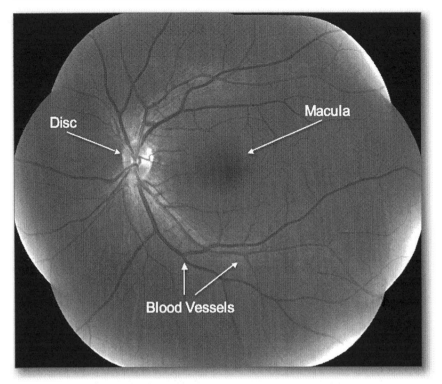

Figure 4: The retina as viewed by your doctor through an ophthalmo-scope. This is the left eye. The right eye would have the macula on the other side of the disc.

Macula

The area of the retina that we pay particular attention to is the *macula*. In Latin, macula means "spot." When the first doctors figured out how to look into the eye, they saw this area of the retina that was dark, and not knowing why it was there, they simply named it "the spot" or the macula. Since then, we've discovered its function. In many ways it is the most important part of the retina because it is the area of your retina that is involved with producing your sharpest clearest vision. The very center of the macula has a special name, the *fovea* or *fovea centralis*. And it is at the fovea where the most detailed vision takes place.

The fovea has a very special architecture. Earlier I described the layers of the retina and the light traveling through all those layers to reach the rods and cones. But those layers can interfere a bit with the light getting to the rods and cones. So, in the fovea, where it is important for the light to get to the cones without any interference, the other layers are pushed out of the way. At the fovea, the light reaches the cones without having to pass through other retinal layers. This area of the retina is thinner, and has a bit of a dip in its contour, like a valley. This dip, or *foveal depression*, is a landmark of the fovea. When we look at diabetic retinopathy, we want to know how close the damage is to your fovea, the center of the macula, because the fovea is responsible for producing your clearest vision.

The center of the macula is what you use for your "straight-ahead" vision, that is, when you're looking directly at something. The rest of the retina can also see, but not as clearly as your fovea. For example, when you look at these words, you are viewing them, one at a time, with your fovea. As you move your eye across the page, you are moving your fovea across each word. Any word that you look at directly is crystal clear, but the words just to the left or right of it are not as clear because those adjacent words are not on the center of the macula. While reading this page, you may also see your hands holding the book; maybe you can see some other things in the room beyond the book. But those objects do not look clear until you move them onto your fovea by looking directly at them. The macula, and its center, the fovea, are for your straight-ahead, sharpest clearest vision. The parts of the retina adjacent to the macula are responsible for your side, or "peripheral" vision, which although very important, do not produce the same clarity as the macula and fovea.

These are the features of the landscape of your retina: the round optic disc and its central optic cup; the blood vessels that emerge from the nerve and branch out to carry blood to the far reaches of the retina; and the macula, with its center, the fovea, where your sharpest clearest vision takes place. In the next few chapters, you will learn how diabetes can affect each of these parts of the "retina-scape."

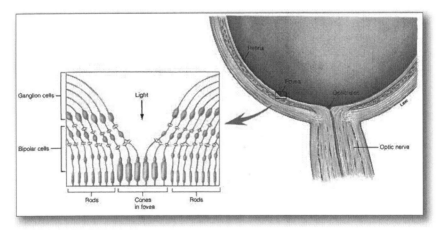

Figure 5: Fovea. The fovea is the very center of the macula, and is where your sharpest clearest vision comes from. At the fovea, the light strikes the cones directly. (This drawing shows the layers of the retina in less detail than Figure 3.)

4

DIABETIC RETINOPATHY: THE EARLY STAGES

Every second, an incredible number of chemical reactions take place within your retina. You can imagine that the retina needs a steady supply of oxygen and nutrients to support these reactions. A constant flow of blood is crucial to keep the retina alive and healthy. When diabetes damages blood vessels, it interferes with oxygen delivery to the retina, resulting in cell damage. The cell damage causes changes in the structure and function of the retina, which can lead to vision loss. We call this damage to the retina *retinopathy*. Because the retina is rich in blood vessels, and diabetes damages blood vessels, the retina is the part of the eye that is damaged most frequently from diabetes. Although diabetes can affect other structures of the eye, when we say "diabetic eye disease," we usually mean diabetic retinopathy.

Types of Diabetic Retinopathy

There are two broad types of diabetic retinopathy. If there are new abnormal blood vessels growing (or "proliferating") inside the eye, we call this *proliferative diabetic retinopathy* (or PDR). This is a severe form of diabetic retinopathy, and I'll discuss PDR in detail in the next chapter.

The early changes that take place, before new abnormal blood vessels grow, are called *non-proliferative diabetic retinopathy* (or NPDR). This form of diabetic retinopathy is commonly called *background diabetic retinopathy* (or BDR). In this chapter, I'll be discussing BDR, which is marked by the following findings:

- microaneurysms
- cotton wool spots
- retinal hemorrhages
- hard exudates
- edema
- venous beading
- IRMA

Microaneurysms

As diabetes begins to damage the blood vessels of the retina, one of the first things that we see are tiny bulges in the blood vessels. These bulges - or *aneurysms* - are the result of the weakening of the blood vessel walls. Because these aneurysms on the retinal blood vessels are so tiny (or "micro") we call them *microaneurysms*. It is the high blood sugar that damages the walls of the blood vessels, causing the weakening and the resultant microaneurysms. These microaneurysms are one of the earliest signs of diabetic retinopathy, and we look carefully for them when we examine your retina. They appear as very fine, almost pinpoint, red dots.

Cotton-wool Spots

In addition to weakening the blood vessel walls, high blood sugar also causes blood vessels to become blocked or occluded. These blockages interfere with oxygen delivery to the superficial layers of the retina. You will recall that when oxygen delivery is compromised, cells and tissues stop working normally. In the retina, the loss of blood flow to the superficial layers of the retina results in swelling, and sometimes even death, of the nerves in that area. The medical term for this loss of blood flow is *ischemia*. The areas of ischemia have soft feathery edges, and are yellow-white in color, in contrast to the red or orange appearance of the healthy retina.

These fluffy yellow-white areas of ischemic retina look a bit like cotton, or wool, and for this reason we call them *cotton-wool spots*. They represent areas of the retina that are not receiving enough oxygen and are not functioning properly. For this reason, I tell my patients that these cotton-wool spots are like tiny strokes within the eye.

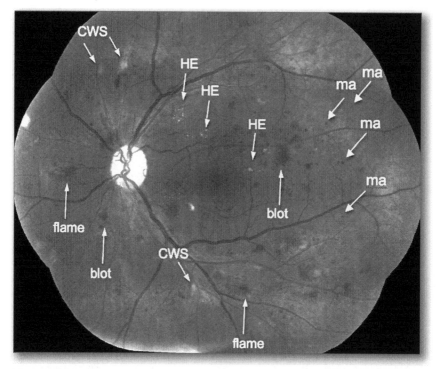

Figure 6: Background diabetic retinopathy. This photo demonstrates many of the findings of diabetic retinopathy. Microaneurysms (ma) appear as small dark dots that are smaller than the diameter of the blood vessels. Cotton-wool spots (CWS) are seen as lighter areas with diffuse edges. There are extensive retinal hemorrhages (flame and blot). The fine lighter areas are hard exudates (HE).

Retinal Hemorrhages

As the high blood sugar continues to damage the blood vessels, the diabetic retinopathy gets worse. Microaneurysms can burst, and other areas of blood vessels can break. When this happens, blood leaks into the surrounding retina, and

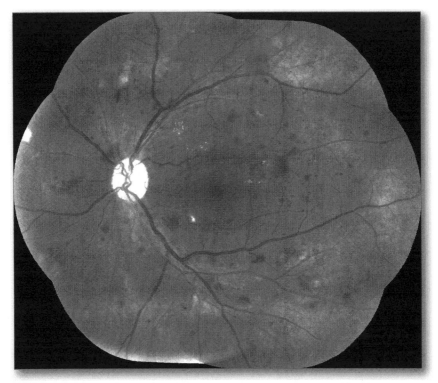

Figure 7: Background diabetic retinopathy. Here is the same photo as in Figure 6, without the labels. Can you identify the findings?

we can see these areas of bleeding when we examine your eyes. We call them *retinal hemorrhages*. If the hemorrhages are in the superficial layers of the retina, they have feathery edges, and we call them *flame* hemorrhages. If they are deeper in the retina, they look more discrete, and we call them *dot* or *blot* hemorrhages. The names describe the amount of bleeding. Blot hemorrhages are bigger than dot hemorrhages, which in turn are bigger than microaneurysms.

Hard Exudates & Edema

In addition to blood leaking out of these damaged blood vessels, fats and proteins can also leak out. Unlike blood, which appears bright red, the proteins and fats are yellow and glistening. We call them *hard exudates*.

Sometimes the blood vessels don't leak blood, proteins or fats. Sometimes they leak only fluid. The fluid itself may be invisible, but it causes swelling or thickening of the retina. We can see this thickening as an elevated area when we examine your retina, and we call this *edema*. Hard exudates and edema are most important when they affect the macula, and especially when they get close to the fovea. Why? Because it is there, at the center of the macula, that hard exudates and edema can have the greatest effect on your vision.

Venous Beading

When non-proliferative diabetic retinopathy becomes severe – that is, when the damage to the blood vessels has become so extensive that there is a severe lack of oxygen – we see two changes that are hallmarks of severe damage. The first is *venous beading*. The retinal veins, instead of having a smooth contour, begin to get a bit lumpy. Some areas of the veins get narrow while other areas appear wider. This can begin to look like a string of sausages, or a string of beads, with alternating narrow and wide areas. Because this can have the same contour as a string of beads, we say that the veins are "beaded."

IRMA

The second change associated with severe non-proliferative diabetic retinopathy is IRMA, which we pronounce just like the woman's name, Irma. The letters stand for *intra-retinal microvascular abnormalities*. As the name describes, tiny blood vessels within the retina become abnormal in shape. Most often, IRMA looks like unusual loops or a squiggly pattern of vessels. Venous beading and IRMA are both signs of severe lack of oxygen. When we see them, we become concerned that danger, which can threaten your vision, is soon to follow.

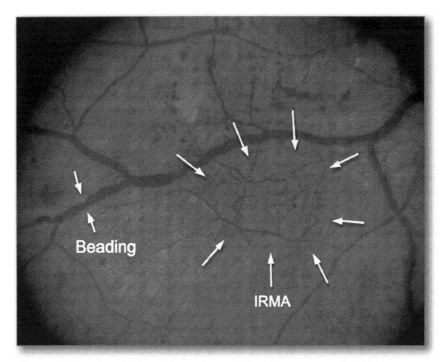

Figure 8: A vein with beading, along with a large area of IRMA.

Classification & Follow-up for BDR

I opened this chapter by explaining that diabetic retinopathy is classified into two broad categories, based on the presence or absence of new abnormal blood vessels: proliferative and non-proliferative ("background") diabetic retinopathy. So far I have discussed the common findings of background diabetic retinopathy. We can further classify background diabetic retinopathy based on its severity. It is important for us to determine the severity of the retinopathy because the severity determines how soon we will need to see you again. The more severe the retinopathy, the more dangerous it is, and the sooner we will need to examine you.

We classify background diabetic retinopathy into four broad categories: mild, moderate, severe, and very severe. We base these categories on the extent of the changes we see. The findings I've described - microaneurysms, cotton-wool spots, flame, and dot and blot hemorrhages, hard exudates, venous beading and IRMA — can occur in any combination. The more of these findings that are present, and the more areas of the retina that are affected, the more severe the retinopathy.

Mild

In mild background diabetic retinopathy, we see only microaneurysms. In such eyes there is little risk to the vision. Typically, in mild diabetic retinopathy, we'll recommend follow-up in one year.

Moderate

If you start to develop cotton-wool spots, retinal hemorrhages, and hard exudates, we classify this as moderate background diabetic retinopathy. This is a broad category, and some of us further sub-classify this category based on how extensive the findings are. Are there just a few retinal hemorrhages? Or are there also lots of hard exudates? Are they limited to one area of the retina, or present throughout the retina? Because of these differences, we may recommend the follow-up visit to be scheduled anywhere from two to six months, depending on what we find during your examination.

Severe

Severe background diabetic retinopathy is designated when we see a specific set of findings. When we look at the retina, we divide the retina into four quadrants, centered on the optic disc. If you have more than twenty retinal hemorrhages in each of the four quadrants, we designate this as severe diabetic retinopathy. Or, if you have venous beading in two quadrants, you have severe diabetic retinopathy. Or, if you have IRMA in one quadrant, we also call this severe diabetic retinopathy. This is called the "4:2:1" rule. More than twenty intra-retinal hemorrhages in four quadrants, or venous beading in two quadrants, or IRMA in one quadrant defines "severe" diabetic retinopathy. With severe diabetic retinopathy, we may recommend follow-up in one to four months.

Very Severe

Very severe background diabetic retinopathy is also defined by the 4:2:1 rule. For severe diabetic retinopathy, you just need one of each of the 4:2:1 findings. But if you have two or more of the 4:2:1 findings, we consider this to be very severe diabetic retinopathy. For example, if you have more than twenty intra-retinal hemorrhages in four quadrants, *and* venous beading in two quadrants, you have very severe diabetic retinopathy.

Sometimes we also call this *pre-proliferative diabetic retinopathy*. By calling it "pre" proliferative, we are indicating that although it is still in a non-proliferative phase, the retinopathy is so severe that new abnormal blood vessels are expected to develop very soon, moving it into the proliferative phase. We want to watch this very closely with follow-up exams as frequently as every one or two months. Sometimes, depending on the circumstances, we may treat very severe non-proliferative diabetic retinopathy as if it were already proliferative diabetic retinopathy.

Importance of Severity

So, the severity of the retinopathy determines how soon we need to see you again. But why? What's so bad about having exudates, intra-retinal hemorrhages, cotton wool spots, or venous beading? In and of themselves, they do not necessarily threaten vision. But, they are signs of the potential development of two vision threatening problems in diabetic retinopathy: macular edema, and proliferative diabetic retinopathy, the subjects of the next two chapters.

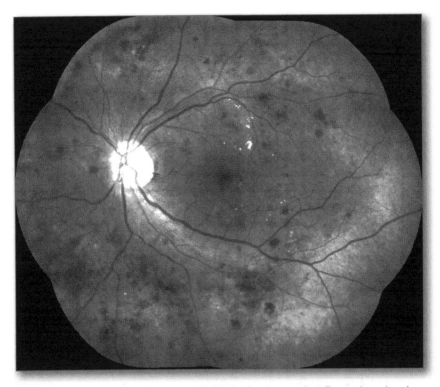

Figure 9: Severe Background Diabetic Retinopathy. Based on having more than twenty retinal hemorrhages in each of the four quadrants centered around the optic disc, this eye would be classified as having severe background diabetic retinopathy. (Also, note the prominent hard exudates above the macula.)

5

MACULAR
EDEMA

You may remember that the most critical part of the retina is the macula, and that the fovea, the very center of the macula, produces your sharpest clearest vision. When we examine your eyes, we give special attention to the macula and the fovea.

When I discuss diabetic retinopathy with my patients, I show them a photograph of their own retina, and I point to the retinal hemorrhages, exudates and areas of swelling throughout the retina, and emphasize that I'm generally not worried about these findings because they are not harmful to the vision. They may look bad, and they may influence how soon I want to see you again, but in and of themselves, the findings of background diabetic retinopathy don't affect vision.

However, if those findings are close to the macula, it's a whole different story. If they are close to the center of the macula, the fovea, they can knock out your vision. So, more than anything else, the location of these findings – how close they are to the fovea — determines how concerned we are about them.

Swelling Leads to Poor Function

A general feature of diabetic retinopathy is leakage of the blood vessels. When the blood vessels first weaken, they develop the bulges and out-pouchings that we call microaneurysms. If the blood vessels leak blood, we see retinal hemorrhages. If they leak protein and fat, we see hard exudates. And if they leak fluid, we see this fluid as swelling or edema of the retina. These leaks, and the swelling that can accompany them, disrupt the delicate layers of the retina and interfere with the ability of the photoreceptors to change light into an electrical signal, and for that electrical signal to get transmitted to your brain. You experience these problems with the photoreceptors and signal transmission as poor vision.

Poor Function Near the Macula Leads to Poor Vision

Anywhere that leakage occurs, it interferes to some degree with the function of the retina, but you won't notice that poor function because most of your retina is not involved with your sharpest clearest vision. However, when that leakage occurs at the center of your macula, it does interfere with your ability to see. Macular edema is the leading cause of vision loss in diabetic eye disease, and most of the treatment we give for diabetic retinopathy is targeted to treating macular edema.

During a retinal exam, much of our time is spent looking at the macula. How much hemorrhage is there? What is the pattern of the exudates in the macula? Do the exudates have swelling near them? And how close are all of these to the center of the macula, the fovea? If the swelling involves the fovea, your vision will likely be blurred, and you will need treatment.

A Silent Threat

Many times the swelling has not yet reached the center of the macula, but is getting very close to it. In this situation, your vision may currently be perfect, nevertheless it may be severely threatened, and you many need treatment. This, in fact, is one of the most dangerous situations you will face. Why? Because your vision will be perfectly fine, yet we'll look into your eye and see a tsunami of edema about to strike the center of your macula. We'll tell you that we need to watch your retina closely, or maybe even treat you to protect your vision — to reverse the tsunami that is bearing down on your fovea. And you are likely to say, "What tsunami? I can see perfectly fine!"

It is this silent, sneaky nature of diabetic retinopathy that results in vision loss. Damage can be occurring without you knowing it or feeling it. A tsunami can be forming that will wipe out your vision, and you're not even aware of it. This is why the eye exam is of such vital importance. It is the only

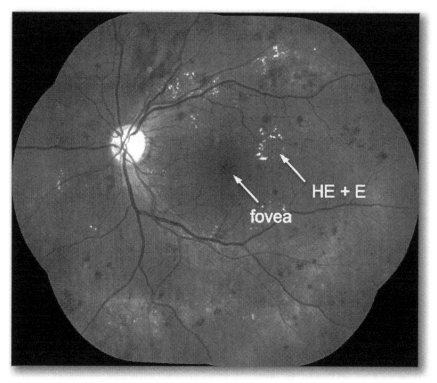

Figure 10: Macular edema. A ring of hard exudates and edema (HE + E) is nearing the fovea, the center of the macula. Although the vision has not yet been affected, you can see that the swelling is getting close to the fovea and that the vision may soon be threatened. Also visible in this photo are scattered retinal hemorrhages, microaneurysms and hard exudates.

way to find out if a tsunami is developing. Even if you don't have blurred vision, diabetic retinopathy may be threatening your vision right now as you read this.

Macular Ischemia

There is another type of damage to the macula that can occur: macular ischemia. Earlier I described that when damage to the blood vessels results in blockage of the blood vessels and loss of blood flow, we call that ischemia. In most of the retina, small areas of ischemia appear as cotton-wool spots. But when blood flow to the center of the macula is compromised, cotton-wool spots don't form, because the center of the macula has a very special architecture and it does not contain the retinal layer where cotton-wool spots would form. In fact, if ischemia occurs at the center of the macula, when we look into your eye, we may not observe anything abnormal at all. But, because there is no blood flow and no oxygen delivery, the cells of the macula that are required for the sharpest clearest vision die, and you experience vision loss.

If you experience vision loss, and we see no macular edema or anything else to explain the poor vision, we suspect that it is due to macular ischemia. We can confirm our suspicion by performing a special test called a fluorescein angiogram that looks at the blood flow through the retina. I'll discuss this test in Chapter 12.

Like macular edema, macular ischemia can occur in people with either non-proliferative or proliferative diabetic retinopathy. But generally, macular ischemia occurs in fairly sick eyes – in people with uncontrolled diabetes with a lot of damage to their blood vessels. Most of the time, the vision loss from macular ischemia is permanent, and there is no treatment available. Preventing macular ischemia is directly related to controlling your blood sugar.

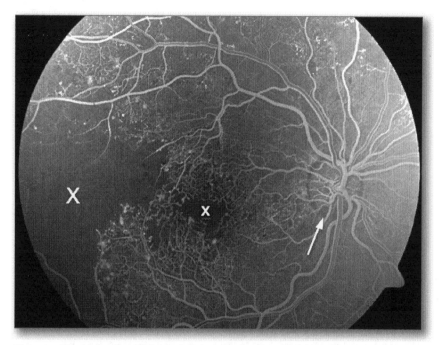

Figure 11: Macular ischemia. A fluorescein angiogram of the right eye shows macular ischemia. The arrow points to the disc. The blood vessels are filled with fluorescein, which allows us to see many of the small blood vessels, the capillaries, which cannot be seen in a retinal photo or during an eye exam. The small "x" marks the macula, which is black, indicating that blood is not flowing in this area. There is also another large area of absent blood flow present to the left of the macula, marked by the large "X." The ischemia in this area does not affect the macula or vision, but it shows that lots of blood vessels have been damaged and the retina is very sick.

6

PROLIFERATIVE DIABETIC RETINOPATHY: NEW BLOOD VESSELS

M acular edema is the leading cause of vision loss in diabetes. The second is proliferative diabetic retinopathy.

From Non-Proliferative to Proliferative

When oxygen delivery to the retina becomes very poor, here is what happens. High blood sugar has already resulted in damage to the blood vessels of the retina. Microaneurysms, retinal hemorrhages, hard exudates, and edema are present. You may have some cotton-wool spots, maybe even some venous beading, or IRMA. But the retinopathy may never get any worse than these background changes. These non-proliferative changes may remain stable and may never threaten your vision. You may have background diabetic retinopathy your whole life, and it may never develop into macular edema or threaten your vision in any way.

But, in some people, particularly those whose blood sugar is high for many years, oxygen delivery to the eye becomes so limited that a strange thing starts to happen in the retina: new blood vessels start to grow. The growth or proliferation of these blood vessels gives this type of diabetic eye disease its name: *proliferative* diabetic retinopathy.

"Neovascularization"

When we examine the retina, we look for the growth of these new blood vessels. We call the growth of new blood vessels, *neovascularization* – *neo* means "new," and *vascular* means "blood vessels." If we see new blood vessels growing on the optic disc, we call this *neovascularization of the disc* or by its abbreviation, *NVD*. We may also find neovascularization in other parts of the retina and we call this *neovascularization elsewhere* or *NVE*. There are special dangers associated with these new blood vessels.

Why Does This Happen?

When high blood sugar damages retinal blood vessels, oxygen delivery is compromised. You already know this. The lack of oxygen has caused the non-proliferative changes. If you are able to control your blood sugar, more damage

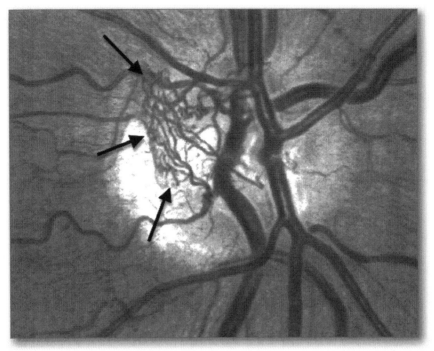

Figure 12: Neovascularization of the disc (NVD). Arrows point to a tangle of new blood vessels, neovascularization, on the surface of the disc.

will not necessarily occur. In fact, tightly controlling your blood sugar can reverse the damage, and result in less diabetic retinopathy.

But if your blood sugar is uncontrolled, or if it is not under excellent control for many years, the damage to the retina can accelerate. I tell my patients that at some point, the retina may become so deprived of oxygen that the retina decides it needs to grow more blood vessels to bring more oxygen to the eye. It is as if the retina is saying, "These old blood vessels

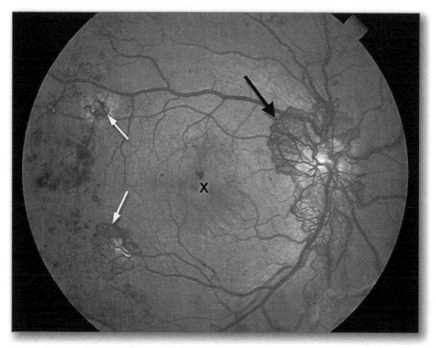

Figure 13: Combined NVD and NVE. Lots of neovascularization (black arrow) covers the disc and has spread to the surrounding retina. Areas of neovascularization elsewhere are marked by the white arrows. Although not related to the neovascularization, the macula (x) has a retinal hemorrhage and appears to be swollen.

are so damaged that they can't bring enough oxygen to my cells. I'm going to grow some new blood vessels." The oxygen-deprived retinal cells send a signal that stimulates the growth of new blood vessels, and that's why the new blood vessels grow. (This signal is called *VEGF* and I'll talk about it in detail in Chapter 18.)

Three Dangers of Neovascularization

But there is a problem. These new blood vessels are not healthy blood vessels. They don't deliver oxygen well. They are very fragile, and they often grow in a disorganized tangle. Often they don't even grow on the surface of the retina, but instead they grow into the vitreous. The new blood vessels are dangerous because they are a threat to your vision. These new blood vessels threaten vision in three major ways: they can easily rupture, filling the eye with blood (*vitreous hemorrhage*); they can contract, putting traction on the retina, causing the retina to detach (*tractional retinal detachment*); and they can block the drainage system of the eye, causing the pressure inside the eye to rise dangerously high (*neovascular glaucoma*). Let's look at each of these.

Threat to Your Vision: Vitreous Hemorrhage

The normal retinal blood vessels are imbedded within the layers of your retina. So when normal retinal blood vessels bleed, as they do in background diabetic retinopathy, the bleeding is usually just a tiny amount, contained within the layers of the retina – the intra-retinal hemorrhages you are familiar with. However, the new dangerous blood vessels in proliferative diabetic retinopathy are located on the surface of the retina, and often extend into the vitreous. So when they rupture, the blood spews into the vitreous, filling the vitreous chamber with blood. You'll recall that the vitreous chamber is that large clear space that makes up most of the eyeball, and lies behind the lens and in front of the retina. Blood in the vitreous chamber blocks light from reaching the retina, and in this way, blocks the vision. We call this kind of bleeding *vitreous hemorrhage*.

Because these blood vessels break suddenly and pour blood into the vitreous chamber, you may actually witness your own vitreous hemorrhage as it happens. You may notice that one minute your vision is fine, and the next you see a sudden shower of floaters, which may, within a few minutes, completely block your vision. Some of my patients tell me that it's as if their vision "turned red," which makes sense, since the light is now being filtered through the red blood in the vitreous.

Sometimes, the bleeding may not spread throughout the entire vitreous. Instead, it may remain localized to a particular part of the vitreous. In these cases, you experience the sensation that something is blocking just a portion of your vision. Some people describe this as clumps in their vision, or spider-webs that float around.

In other cases, the blood may not extend into the vitreous at all, but may remain just in front of the retina, wedged between the surface of the retina and the back of the vitreous. This kind of bleeding is called *pre-retinal hemorrhage* ("pre" because it lies immediately in front of the retina). Sometimes, a localized vitreous hemorrhage or pre-retinal hemorrhage may occur far from your macula, and you may not have any symptoms at all.

Three things determine if a vitreous hemorrhage will affect your vision: where it is, how big it is, and whether it's localized or diffuse. If a vitreous hemorrhage is over the macula or close to the macula, you're probably going to notice it and

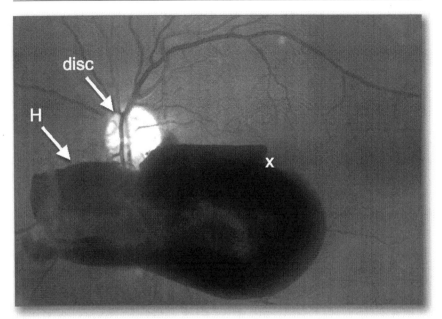

Figure 14: Pre-retinal hemorrhage. A large pre-retinal hemorrhage (H) below the disc and over part of the macula (x) of the left eye. The hemorrhage blocks the underlying retina, but note that the view of the retina in other places is clear. This is because the hemorrhage is wedged between the back of the vitreous and the surface of the retina, and has not spread into the vitreous.

it will affect your vision. But if it is far from the macula, in the periphery, you may not know that you've had a vitreous hemorrhage. However, if it is in the periphery, and really big, you may notice it as a cloud or curtain over part of your vision. On the other hand, no matter where the hemorrhage starts, if it spreads throughout your vitreous (that is, if it is diffuse), then it will cause a haze and will affect your vision.

I share this with you because you may end up having more than one vitreous hemorrhage over time. These hemorrhages don't all behave the same. Sometimes you'll notice them, but sometimes only your doctor will be able to see them. Sometimes they'll interfere with your vision, and sometimes they won't. But despite these differences, any vitreous hemorrhage is a sign that neovascularization is present, which puts you

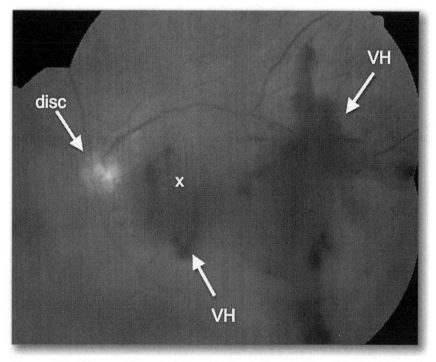

Figure 15: Vitreous hemorrhage in the left eye. The disc and lower part of the retina are not clearly visible because of diffuse blood in that part of the vitreous. The retina at the top appears clearer because there is not much blood in that part of the vitreous. To the right of the disc, a large dense vitreous hemorrhage (VH) appears as a dark splotch blocking our view of the underlying retina. This kind of vitreous hemorrhage can cause sudden decrease in your vision, because light cannot reach the macula (x) through the blood.

at higher risk for eventual vision loss. So generally, treatment is needed when a vitreous hemorrhage occurs.

Unfortunately, many people go to an eye specialist for the first time when they experience a large vitreous hemorrhage. This is not a good thing. It means that for years the diabetic retinopathy has been progressing from mild to moderate to severe, completely unnoticed. The opportunity to get treatment early has been lost because there were no eye exams. If the new abnormal blood vessels are spotted before the vitreous hemorrhage happens, we can treat them and prevent the bleeding.

Threat to Your Vision: Tractional Retinal Detachment

The second way that these new blood vessels threaten your vision is by tugging on and wrinkling your retina. Often the new blood vessels are accompanied by fibrous elements that can contract. We refer to this combination of fibrous elements and new blood vessels as *fibrovascular* changes. As the fibrovascular elements contract, they tug on the surrounding retina, causing the retina to move from its normal position. The retina lifts away from its normal position on the sclera and become *detached*. These detachments are caused by traction, so we call them *tractional retinal detachments*.

A tractional retinal detachment is usually limited to a small area of the retina. Just as with edema, if the tractional retinal detachment does not involve the center of the macula, it may not affect your vision. In many cases the tractional detachment can be left alone and observed. But if it begins to tug on the macula, it can affect your vision. If the macula is detached, vision can be lost. In some cases, tractional retinal detachments can become so severe that the whole retina detaches and gets crumpled up like a wad of paper, resulting in total loss of vision. Tractional retinal detachments can be fixed, but the more of the retina that gets crumpled up, the more difficult it is to repair. Often, with severe detachments,

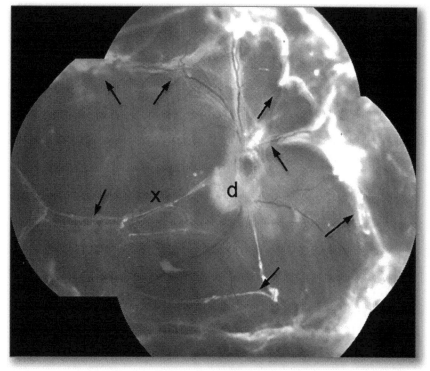

Figure 16: Extensive fibrovascular tissue and tractional retinal detachments (arrows). The white bands are a combination of fibrovascular tissue and elevation of the retina. The disc (d) is mostly covered with white fibrous tissue, and the macula (x) has traction extending across it.

we may be able to re-attach the retina, but the vision may not improve.

It's important to monitor things so that the detachments do not become severe. You may have a tractional retinal detachment right now that is not causing any symptoms, yet it may be threatening your macula, or putting your whole retina and your vision at risk. Again, this emphasizes the need to get your eyes examined and to keep your follow-up appointments. There is much we can do to prevent blindness from proliferative diabetic retinopathy, but only if you are getting your eyes examined regularly.

Threat to Your Vision: Neovascular Glaucoma

NVD and NVE both refer to new blood vessels growing in the back of the eye – on the disc and elsewhere on the retina. However, there is another place that neovascularization can occur: in the front part of the eye, on the iris. We call this, *neovascularization of the iris* or *NVI*. The new blood vessels are growing on the iris, not because the iris is sick, but because the retina is sick – really sick. Think of it in this way: the retina is so ischemic that its distress signals are not only causing NVD and NVE in the back of the eye, but they're also reaching the front of the eye, causing the iris to grow new blood vessels too.

No matter where they occur, new blood vessels are a sign of a very sick retina, and the risk of permanent vision loss is particularly high. But when NVI develops, it is an emergency because it can cause permanent blindness in a matter of days. Recent advances in treatment have made it possible to save the vision, but like everything else I've talked about, it depends upon early diagnosis and treatment.

To understand how NVI can result in such rapid loss of vision, I need to give you a little bit more information on the inner workings of the eye. The eye is a ball, and like any ball, it has a certain pressure inside it. If the pressure inside the eye is too high, the structures inside the eye can get damaged from the high pressure.

The pressure inside the eye is determined by the balance between the fluid that is being formed inside the eye, and the fluid leaving the eye. In the deeper parts of the eye, a structure called the *ciliary body* constantly produces a fluid, called *aqueous humor*, which helps maintain the pressure of the eye and provides nutrients to the structures of the eye. As the fluid is being produced, it is also being drained from the eye, in an area called the *trabecular meshwork*. It is this balance between the production of fluid by the ciliary body, and the drainage of fluid through the trabecular meshwork, that determines the pressure inside the eye. If the drain, the trabecular meshwork, becomes clogged or sealed, the fluid builds up inside the eye and causes the pressure to rise.

The trabecular meshwork lies in the angle where the iris meets the cornea. The new blood vessels that grow on the iris have easy access to the trabecular meshwork, and can creep onto the meshwork and seal it up. Once it's sealed, the pressure shoots up to dangerously high levels. When the pressure rises and does damage to the structures of the eye because of NVI, we call this *neovascular glaucoma*. In fact, with NVI, the pressure can rise to dangerously high levels and lead to total blindness in a matter of days. It can be extremely painful, and the damage to vision is usually permanent. During every exam, we check carefully for NVI. If it is present, we act quickly to get rid of it. Sometimes we are successful, but sometimes irreversible damage has already been done.

By now you may have realized that the reason diabetes can be so devastating is because so much of the damage happens without you knowing about it. It is silent. You can't feel it. You may have had diabetes for years and still have great vision. But the damage is occurring, quietly, sneakily, without you knowing it. The damage may be getting close to snuffing out your sight, either through macular edema, vitreous hemorrhage, tractional retinal detachment or neovascular glaucoma, while you go about your life, unaware of the diabetic retinopathy raging inside your eyes.

I tell my patients that the most common, and most dangerous symptom of diabetic eye disease is that there are no symptoms. Because there are no symptoms, you think that nothing is wrong, and therefore you don't bother getting an eye exam. Now you understand how diabetic eye disease causes damage, and how it can rob you of your sight. You know that the only way to catch the problems early is to have a complete eye exam by an eye specialist.

If there is one message I hope you take from this first section, it is this: an eye exam every year is the first step toward saving your vision. If we see the problems, we can treat them and save your sight. If you don't give us the chance to check you, diabetic retinopathy can do its damage hidden from us, causing permanent loss of your vision. If you haven't had an eye exam in the past year, or if you missed your appointment, this is a good time to pick up the phone and schedule an appointment.

Let's now turn to a few other problems that can affect your vision in diabetes.

7

CATARACTS

You'll recall that in order to see properly, light has to enter the eye, pass through the cornea, the pupil, and the lens, and land on the retina. If anything interferes with the passage of light through these structures, vision is compromised.

Sometimes, the lens inside the eye can become cloudy. We call a cloudy lens a *cataract*. When the lens becomes cloudy, light cannot pass into the eye very well. It's a bit like the window of a house or car getting cloudy or foggy. You just can't see well through the cloudy window. In the same way, cataracts interfere with your ability to see clearly.

Cataracts are a natural part of aging. If you live long enough, you'll likely end up with cataracts. However, in diabetes, cataracts tend to develop at a younger age. If you don't have diabetes you'll probably develop cataracts sometime after you turn 60 or 70. If you get diabetes at an early age, it's not uncommon to develop cataracts in your 40's and 50's.

Types of Cataracts

Different parts of the lens can get cloudy. The lens can get cloudy at the edges or in the center. It can get cloudy in the front, the middle or the back. The cloudiness can be the result of increased density of the lens, opacities of the lens, or changes in color in the lens. The cloudiness can be partial or total. When we examine your lens, we describe these changes. We use words like "nuclear sclerosis," "posterior subcapsular cataracts," "anterior cortical cataracts," and "brunescent cataracts" to describe the specific pattern of changes in your lens.

It's not so important for you to know the specifics of each of these types of cataracts. Rather, by knowing that there are different types of cataracts, you can understand why different people have different symptoms from cataracts. For example, some type of cataracts simply cause your vision to blur, others cause you to see the world through a yellow tint, while

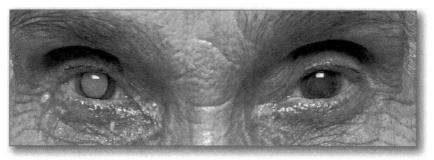

Figure 17: A person with a very cloudy lens – a total cataract — in the right eye. The white cloudy lens is easy to see through the dilated pupil. The left eye has a slight cataract that is not very noticeable in this photo.

others cause you to be sensitive to bright lights. Some cataracts cause you to experience glare and halos around bright lights, and can make driving at night very difficult. In many people, there are several different types of lens changes occurring together, and so you may experience a combination of these symptoms.

Cataract Surgery is Easy for You

In general, glasses do not remove the symptoms of cataracts; eye drops and pills do not treat cataracts. But there is a good treatment for cataracts, and that is to remove the cloudy lens and replace it with a new clear artificial lens. This is called *cataract surgery.*

Most of the time, when we say "surgery," people get scared. That's normal. Someday, I'll need cataract surgery, and even though I've done the surgery thousands of times and know how safe it is, I expect even I will be a bit scared too. To calm my patients' fears, I explain how, for you, as a patient, the operation is easy. And by "easy" I mean that it is quick, painless, and doesn't disrupt your life significantly.

For the surgery, you come in, you have the surgery, and you go home the same day. The surgery takes about fifteen minutes. We make your eye numb, so there is no pain, and we give you some medication to help you relax. Most people take a nap during the surgery.

After the surgery, we put a clear cover over your eye, which allows you to see through the eye immediately after surgery. And we give you eye drops to use at home that day. By the next day, most people return to work or are back to their regular activities. In this sense the recovery is very quick, but you will use eye drops for about a month to help the eye fully heal. And during this time, we will check you regularly — usually the day after surgery, a week after surgery, and a month after surgery. At that one-month visit, most people find that an update in their eyeglass prescription will fine-tune their vision.

Are There Restrictions After Surgery?

Maybe you remember a parent or grandparent having cataract surgery years ago, and being told that they couldn't engage in their regular activities for several weeks – no bending, no lifting, no straining, things like that. You may wonder if you'll have similar restrictions. The answer, generally, is no. You can return to your regular activities right after surgery. How can this be?

Modern cataract surgery techniques make the procedure minimally invasive and minimally disruptive. The best surgeons use special instruments that allow us to remove the cataract through tiny incisions that are self-sealing, and rarely require sutures. The development of modern cataract surgery has been a quest for smaller and smaller incisions, and faster and faster recovery times. Instead of removing the cataract as a whole, which requires a large incision and a long healing time, we now use sophisticated machines that gently dissolve the lens, allowing us to remove it through incisions that are less than three millimeters in size. Instead of using a lens implant that goes in through an incision the same size as the lens, we now have implants that we can fold up like a taco, and be inserted through the same tiny incision. Once inside the eye, the lens implant gently unfolds to its full size.

These technologies allow us to make small self-sealing incisions, and it is these small incisions that allow for your rapid recovery. In the old days, when we made larger incisions, we would caution our patients to avoid bending, lifting or straining for several weeks while the large incision healed. Because the modern incision is small and self-sealing, you can go back to your regular activities the day after the surgery, including most sports.

Finally, any artificial lens that is implanted inside the eye is a permanent lens and does not need to be removed or replaced, except under the rarest of circumstances. You can expect to have the same lens implant in your eye for the rest of your life, without the need to remove it.

Safety of Surgery

Despite the ease of surgery for you, and the rapid recovery time, I don't want to give the impression that cataract surgery is "minor" surgery. It is a delicate procedure, requiring a skilled ophthalmologist with steady hands and good judgment to perform the surgery successfully.

Like any surgery (or like anything else in life, really), cataract surgery does have some risks, but the risks of serious complications, such as infection, are small – less than 1/1000.

I always have a detailed discussion of risks with my patients, and I tell them, "I'm not telling you about the risks to make you nervous. I'm telling you about the risks because it's my responsibility as your doctor to make sure you know that, just like everything else in life, there are risks involved. Getting in a car has risks, walking down stairs has risks, and cataract surgery also has risks. The risks are small, but they're there."

We do everything possible to decrease the risks, but we can't make the risks "zero." Throughout this book, I'll discuss various treatments and procedures, and the same principle applies. Everything in life (and in medicine) has risks. And though we can decrease the risks, we cannot eliminate them. The key is to compare the risks of a particular path, with the benefits and alternatives. The benefit of cataract surgery is better vision, and it's a rare person who does not want cataract surgery given the overall safety and success of the surgery.

It is the most commonly preformed surgery in the world, with millions of people benefiting from cataract surgery every year. Your doctor will discuss the risks, benefits and alternatives of cataract surgery (and of any procedure) with you. The ultimate decision about treatment is always yours.

Lens Implant Options

Monofocal and Monovision

When it comes time for your cataract surgery, your doctor may discuss with you the various lens implant options available.

Traditionally, we have used fixed focus, or *monofocal* lens implants. Monofocal means that the focus of the lens is set for one particular distance. Most people like to have their far vision clear, and then use reading glasses for near vision.

Another option that some people choose with monofocal lenses is to have the focus in one eye set for distance and the other eye set for near. We call this *monovision*. With monovision, you can see both distance and near without glasses. My eyes naturally have monovision, and I love it – one of my eyes sees clearly in the distance, but not so well at near; the other is nearsighted – I can see things up close clearly with it, but not in the distance. So, in every day life, I can get by without glasses because I can see the distance with one eye, and near with the other eye. I do have a pair of glasses that I wear when I want to really sharpen things up in both eyes, like when I'm reading for a long period of time, or going to the movies. But day-to-day, I get along fine without glasses. Monovision isn't for everyone, but it's a consideration if you want to use monofocal lenses.

The advantages of monofocal lenses are that the cost of the lenses is usually covered by Medicare and by other medical insurance plans, and that they are straightforward lenses to use. The disadvantage is that they are only set for one distance, so unless you get monovision, you'll need to wear glasses for reading and other close work every day.

Presbyopia Correcting Lens Implants

When most of us hit age forty, we're afflicted by one of nature's cruelties: we lose the ability to see up close and so we need to wear reading glasses. This condition, the inability to focus up close, is called *presbyopia*, which means "old vision." Your natural lens, which is flexible during your youth, can change its focus to allow you to see distance and near. But as you get older, the lens loses its flexibility and with it, its ability to focus up close. When presbyopia first sets in around age forty, you'll notice that the closer you hold something, the blurrier it gets. You can compensate for a while simply by holding things farther away to bring them into focus. But you'll soon find that your arms aren't long enough to hold things as far as you need to hold them to get them into focus. And so, you get your first pair of reading glasses or bifocals. We've been trying to solve the problem of presbyopia for years – to come up with some treatment to avoid the inconvenience of reading glasses. Although we haven't found an easy way to fix presbyopia, we have come up with a way to get rid of presbyopia at the time of cataract surgery.

When we replace your cataract with a monofocal lens, that lens implant, like your natural forty-plus year-old lens, is stiff and cannot focus far and near at the same time. Wouldn't it be great if we could develop a lens implant that could return your youthful vision, solve the problems of presbyopia, and give you the ability to see distance and near without reading glasses, and without monovision? For many years we worked on solving this problem, and during the first decade of the twenty-first century, we finally came up with the technology to make lens implants that could reliably give good near and distance vision. We call these *presbyopia correcting lens implants*.

Two Kinds of Presbyopia Correcting Implants

There are two major categories of presbyopia correcting lens implants that allow this type of youthful vision. One category either has a hinge on it or is made of very soft material, which allows the lens to have a bit of flexibility, just like your natural youthful lens. These lens implants are able to shift a bit when you try to view near objects, and by shifting, they bring near objects into focus.

The other type of lens implant is the multifocal lens. The multifocal lens, although not flexible, is designed with different areas of focus within the lens to allow for simultaneous near and distance vision. It focuses near and distance images all at the same time, and your brain naturally chooses which image it wants to pay attention to. Usually, both eyes need to have the surgery within a few weeks of one another to get the best results. Occasionally, your vision is not as sharp as expected, and you will need additional surgical adjustments to fine-tune the focus.

Each of these types of presbyopia correcting lenses has its limitations, and the lenses are not for everyone. Rarely, some people find that they are unhappy with the presbyopia correcting lenses and have them removed and replaced with monofocal lenses. However, most people love their presbyopia correcting lens implants, because the lenses give them the ability to see at all distances without relying significantly on glasses. Your eye specialist can discuss with you whether or not you are a good candidate for one of these lenses.

The main disadvantage of presbyopia correcting lenses is cost. These lenses are usually not covered by insurance, and they can cost up to several thousand dollars extra per eye. To get the most benefit, both eyes need to have presbyopia correcting lenses implanted.

Diabetes and Cataract Surgery

Many of my patients with diabetes ask me if it's safe for them to have cataract surgery even if they have diabetes. The truth is, most of the people I perform cataract surgery on have

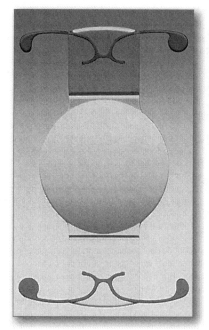 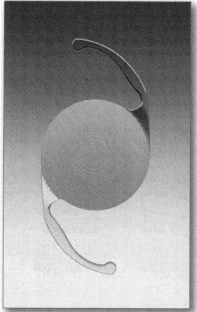

Figure 18: A hinged presbyopia correcting lens, which flexes to allow you to shift your focus between distant and near objects.

Figure 19: A multifocal presbyopia correcting lens has a series of rings on its surface that results in being able to focus at near and far at the same time.

diabetes. If you have diabetes, you can certainly have cataract surgery. Often we will have your family doctor check you to make sure that you are healthy enough for surgery, and that your blood sugar and blood pressure are under good enough control.

For most people with diabetes, cataract surgery results in a dramatic improvement in vision. Replacing the cloudy lens results in perfectly clear vision if all the other parts of the eye are functioning well. But if you have diabetic retinopathy, it is possible that the damage that has already occurred to your retina will limit your vision. For example, if you have macular edema, macular ischemia, or a macular tractional retinal detachment, removing the cataract, though it may improve your vision, may not give you perfect vision. The underlying problems with your macula limit your vision. However, removal of the cataract will give you the clearest vision possible, and if your macula is healthy, you will see well. Your ophthalmologist can advise you on the expected improvement from cataract surgery with your particular level of diabetic retinopathy.

Another consideration is that cataract surgery can have an effect on diabetic retinopathy, sometimes causing it to worsen. Studies have shown that when we give certain drugs (like Avastin – a drug I'll discuss in detail in Chapters 18, 19 and 20) or laser treatment (which I'll discuss in Chapters 15 and 16) before cataract surgery, we can improve the visual outcome and help prevent the worsening of the diabetic retinopathy. We use these treatments to get your retina in the best condition possible as we move toward cataract surgery.

Finally, removal of the cataract has an additional benefit. Sometimes the cataract can be so cloudy that it not only blocks your vision, but also interferes with your doctor's ability to clearly see your retina. And if we can't see your retina, we can't determine the extent of retinopathy or determine if you need treatment. Removing the cataract gives us a clear view of the retina. As a result, we are able to fully evaluate your retina and make recommendations for treatment.

———————

Modern cataract surgery is one of the miracles of medicine. If your vision is limited because of a cataract, this short procedure, with its minimal recovery time, can quickly give you your vision back.

8

FLUCTUATING VISION

O ne of the most frustrating challenges of diabetes is fluctuating vision. Maybe you've experienced this. On some days your vision is better, and on others, it's worse. One day everything is clear, then a few days later it's blurry, then better again. Maybe you have three pairs of glasses — all different prescriptions — and depending on the day of the week, you find that a particular pair works better than the others. And on some days, nothing seems to give you clear vision. What is going on? Why is your vision fluctuating?

Focusing Light

These changes in vision are related to the rise and fall of your blood glucose. Remember that the natural lens inside your eye helps focus images onto your retina. To see clearly, the light has to be perfectly focused on your retina. Some people's eyes are set so that the light focuses perfectly on the retina. But for many people, the cornea and lens don't focus light perfectly onto the retina. These eyes need some extra help getting the image to focus on the retina, and they get this help by placing extra lenses in front of the eyes, either as glasses or contact lenses. These extra lenses make up for the imprecise focusing of the eyes. That's what glasses are all about. Your eyes don't focus the light on the retina so the glasses are made to match your eyes' particular focusing deficiency, and to focus light precisely on the retina.

If you wear glasses, you know that from year to year your eyes' ability to focus may change. That's why every year you get your eye prescription evaluated. Sometimes it changes and you will need new glasses; at other times there's no change in your eyes' focusing ability and therefore no change in your eyeglass prescription. When you have difficulty focusing light, we call this a *refractive error*.

Refractive Errors

There are three main types of refractive errors: *myopia*, commonly called nearsightedness, where the light focuses in front of the retina; *hyperopia*, where the light focuses behind the retina; and *astigmatism*, where the eye, instead of being round like a basketball, is shaped more like a football, which causes different rays of light to focus in different places in relation to the retina. It's possible to have astigmatism in combination with myopia or hyperopia.

It's also possible to have different types of refractive errors in each eye.

Blood Sugar and Focus

With diabetes, instead of your eyes' focusing ability changing over a year or so, changes can occur in a matter of days. How does this happen over such a short period of time? Well, it's all related to the effect that blood sugar has on the shape of your natural lens. Changes in shape of the lens affect its focus. You see, when your blood sugar rises, it causes the natural lens inside your eye to swell a bit. The extra sugar goes into the lens, and it takes water into the lens with it, causing the lens to swell. This shifts the focus of the eye and makes the vision blurry. As your blood sugar goes back down again, the extra sugar leaves your natural lens, and the water leaves with it. The swelling decreases, and the lens then focuses differently, and your vision shifts again.

These changes in the shape of the lens take some time. So if your blood sugar is high for a few hours, and then comes back down to normal levels again, you probably won't notice a change in your vision. But if your blood sugar is high for a few days, you may experience vision changes. These changes are not a sign of permanent damage to your eyes. They are a sign of changes in your blood sugar, which change the shape of your lens and its focusing ability. The treatment of this changing vision is to control the blood sugar, keeping it steady and avoiding wide fluctuations.

Some people know when their blood sugar is high for a few days because they notice a shift in their vision. To see clearly in this situation, a new eyeglass prescription would be needed to match the shift in the refractive error. Should you get a new pair of glasses for these shifts in your blood sugar? Usually we don't recommend it. Instead, we recommend getting your blood sugar under control. We know that if your blood sugar has been running, say, 200, and we prescribe glasses today, when the blood sugar comes down to 120, and your focus shifts again, that particular pair of glasses that we gave you when the blood sugar was running 200 won't be very helpful any more. That pair of glasses is useful only when the blood sugar is around 200.

On the other hand, if your blood sugar never gets down to 120, and you always stay around 200, we may prescribe new glasses for you. Once we know your baseline blood sugar — the blood sugar level on most days - we're okay to prescribe new glasses.

Vision that fluctuates every few days or weeks is often related to changing blood sugar. Like many of the problems with diabetes, the solution lies in controlling your blood sugar. The changes in blood sugar cause changes in the shape of the natural lens in the eye, which cause changes in the focus - the refractive error — of the eye. This explains why different eyeglass prescriptions may work on some days, but not on others. It can be very frustrating.

If you are having symptoms of fluctuating vision, it can be a sign that your blood sugar is fluctuating. Your eye specialist and your general medical doctor can work together to determine the cause and to adjust your diet or medications to better control your blood sugar and put an end to the fluctuating vision.

9

DOUBLE VISION

A small percentage of people with diabetes, at some point over the years, will develop double vision. Some people confuse "double vision" with "blurred vision." What I mean by "double vision" is that you see two of everything. For example, you look at someone's face and you see two faces next to each other. The two faces may be right next to each other — maybe even overlapping; or they may be far apart, like you're looking at twins. The world is double. And if you cover one eye — either eye, it doesn't matter which one — the double vision disappears and you see one of everything. But when you uncover your eye and use both eyes, everything becomes double again.

Two Eyes, One Image

To understand the problem of double vision, I need to explain how the two eyes work together. Each of your eyes sends an image of the world to your brain. However, the images are not exactly the same, because one of your eyes sees the world from a perspective a little to the left of your nose, and the other eye sees the world from a little to the right of your nose. But your eyes are precisely aligned and coordinated so that your brain "sees" only one image. In fact, the very slight difference between the images from each eye is what allows depth perception. It's what allows you to see in three dimensions, or "3-D." (Close one eye during a 3-D movie and the 3-D effect disappears.)

If the images that your two eyes are sending to your brain are not precisely aligned, your brain will not be able to combine the two images into a single 3-D image. Instead, you will see them as two separate images, or "double." Double vision, or *diplopia*, results when anything interferes with the precise alignment of the two eyes. Let me explain.

Muscles and Nerves Control Eye Movement

Under normal circumstances, the movement of each eye is controlled by six muscles. I tell my patients that the muscles around the eye are a little bit like the reins on a horse. If the left rein gets tighter the horse's head will move to the left. In the same way, if the muscle on the left side of the eye tightens (or *contracts*) the eye moves to the left. Around each eye, there are two muscles that move the eye horizontally – to the left and to the right (just like the reins); there are two muscles that move the eye vertically, up and down; and two more muscles that move the eye obliquely, helping you rotate your eyes when you tilt your head, or moving the eyes in diagonal directions. These two horizontal muscles (for left and right movements), the two vertical muscles (for up-and-down movements), and the two oblique muscles (for rotational and diagonal movements) make up the six muscles around each eye.

The six muscles of each eye are in turn controlled by three separate nerves that come from the brain. Each of these nerves starts in the back of the brain, follows a specific path to get to your eye socket, and then attaches to and controls the eye muscle that it's in charge of.

When There Are Problems

But sometimes things can go wrong with this system, and the eyes lose their alignment; then the images don't match up in your brain, and as a result, you have double vision. Things can go wrong in any number of places and for all kinds of reasons. Problems can arise in the brain, where the nerves start; along the path of the nerves where they pass over bone, blood vessels and brain tissue; and in the eye sockets. Sometimes problems can occur with the muscles themselves. And problems can be caused by anything from tumors to aneurysms to fractures, strokes, metabolic diseases, and muscle or nerve conditions. Double vision can be caused by all sorts of things, some of which are quite serious, and some of which are not. Our job, as doctors, is to find the cause of the double vision. Your job is to know that double vision is a reason to see your doctor right away.

Isolated Nerve Palsy

If you have diabetes and you develop double vision, here is what we do. First we check to see which eye muscles and nerves are involved. This can be done by examining the movement of the eyes. Then we check to see if any other nerves that control other parts of the face or body are involved. We pay special attention to your pupils. We check things like the sensation of your face, the movement of your facial muscles, your hearing, and the movements of your tongue and throat. These can all give us clues to what is going on.

If these other areas are all normal and the double vision is caused by a single nerve problem, we call it an "isolated" nerve palsy (*palsy* means "paralysis" or "weakness.") The fact that the double vision is caused by a single nerve tells us that something big and bad, like a tumor or an aneurysm, is probably not the cause. Those things usually affect several nerves at the same time.

If it is not an isolated nerve palsy — for example, if in addition to the misalignment of the eyes your pupil is involved, or your eyelid won't close, or a part of your face is droopy or numb — then we are more concerned. Your body is giving us clues that the problem is affecting several structures and needs more investigation. But the typical problem we see in diabetes is the isolated nerve palsy - one nerve of one eye causes some imbalance of eye movement, resulting in a misalignment of the eyes, which in turn causes a misalignment of the images sent to the brain that are then seen as "double."

Cause of Nerve Palsy in Diabetes

So what causes these isolated nerve palsies in diabetes? You know from our earlier discussions that diabetes causes damage to blood vessels. The damage interferes with the flow of blood and oxygen, and the lack of oxygen damages organs supplied by those blood vessels. The isolated nerve palsies that cause double vision in diabetes are usually caused because not enough blood and oxygen are reaching a nerve. This lack of blood and oxygen causes the nerve to malfunction. The nerve cannot send its signal to the muscle, and so the alignment and coordination between the two eyes get thrown off, resulting in double vision. When the brain malfunctions because of a sudden loss of blood flow, we call it a *stroke*. So this malfunction of a nerve from a loss of blood flow is like a tiny stroke to that nerve.

Prognosis and Treatment

The good news is, usually there is full recovery. With the passage of time, blood flow is reestablished to the nerve, the nerve recovers its function, the eyes get aligned once again, and the double vision goes away. This healing process usually takes six to twelve weeks. Most people make a full recovery. But if the nerve palsy is unusual in some way, or if it lasts longer than expected, then we do additional tests that usually include a CT scan or MRI of the brain to make sure nothing else is going on.

While the nerve palsy is present, the double vision can be very annoying. It can make everyday tasks quite difficult.

Most people will naturally close one eye to get rid of the double vision. Some people decide to wear a patch over the eye to eliminate the double vision, instead of walking around all day with one eye closed. In rare cases a diabetic nerve palsy does not go away, and then special glasses, or sometimes even surgery are needed to align the images and get rid of the double vision.

Since double vision can be caused by many different things, some of them very serious and even life threatening, it's important to see your eye specialist immediately if you develop double vision. If it is from an isolated nerve palsy from diabetes, you can expect that it will recover completely in six to twelve weeks.

PART II

THE

EYE EXAM

In this section, my goal is to remove any anxiety you might have about an eye exam by explaining what happens every step of the way. In the first chapter of this section, I discuss how to prepare for your visit to the doctor. I don't want you to think that there is a lot of preparation to make before you visit the doctor, because there isn't. But by taking a few items with you, it can make things go smoother. If you don't have everything with you, it's not a big deal. If you're able to gather everything, great. If not, don't let it delay your visit to your eye doctor because getting your eyes examined is the first step to saving your vision.

In the second chapter of this section, I go through the eye exam step-by-step. Whether you know these steps or not doesn't affect the care you receive, so again, this is not something for you to worry about. But if you're curious about what is taking place at each step, or if knowledge makes you feel more comfortable, I think you'll find this chapter very useful.

The third chapter explains some of the specialized tests you may receive because of your diabetic eye disease. Eye care, more than almost any other field, takes full advantage of the recent advances in technology to help diagnose and treat disease. Here you'll become familiar with the five most common tests for diabetic retinopathy.

Finally, I spend a short chapter discussing the eye exams that you'll have in the future, and what determines when you will need another eye exam, and what can happen if you miss your follow-up appointments.

10

PREPARING TO SEE THE DOCTOR

A ny time people face the unknown, it is natural to experience anxiety. A few years ago, I was having some neck pain that would not go away. It was so severe that I could not turn my head, and I was in pain all day long. My general doctor could not find an explanation, and nothing improved over several months, so I made an appointment to see a neurosurgeon. On my way to my appointment with the neurosurgeon, I was nervous. I was worried about the diagnosis. What would the doctor find? What if it was something serious? What if I had to have surgery? What if I got paralyzed? What if the pain would not go away and I had to spend the rest of my life like Frankenstein, unable to turn my head? What if young children would run screaming at the sight of me? What if? What if? What if?

All of these thoughts were raging in my head. But when I walked into the doctor's office, a whole new set of anxieties was triggered. I realized that despite being a doctor myself, I had come unprepared. I didn't have pieces of information with me that would make things easier for me and for the doctor. I also realized that I had some anxiety because I didn't know what to expect. How long would I be there? What would the examination be like? What tests might I need?

I made it through the visit but I wish I had been better prepared. I could have avoided the extra anxiety. In this chapter I will give you the information you need to arrive prepared at your doctor's office, and to know what to expect during the visit.

What to Take

When you visit a doctor's office, we need two kinds of information. We need information about you, and we need information about your health. Most of the information you'll know, but things can go faster if you take a few things with you.

First, if you have medical insurance, such as Medicare or Medicaid or private insurance, take your insurance card with you. This helps with the registration process. If you have a form of photo ID, such as a driver's license, take that too.

Next, take either a list of all your medications, or take the medications themselves. Many medications can have an effect on the eyes, and it helps us to know exactly what you are taking even if they are not eye medications.

Also, if you wear eyeglasses or contact lenses, bring your current pair with you. We can measure your glasses to determine the prescription, but we can't do this easily with contact lenses. So please bring your contact lens boxes since the prescription is written on them.

Bring a pair of sunglasses too. Sometimes after an eye exam you may be sensitive to light, and sunglasses will help. If you don't have a pair, the doctor's office can provide you with a disposable pair to get you home. Some people find it too bright to drive home, and bring someone with them to drive.

Finally, take some form of payment. There is usually a co-payment required by your insurance company, and it helps keep expenses down if you are prepared to take care of this co-payment at the time of your visit.

Remember to Take

✓ Insurance Card
✓ Photo ID
✓ Medications
✓ Eyeglasses
✓ Contact lenses with boxes
✓ Sunglasses
✓ Someone to drive you home (if you need this)
✓ Payment

Information About Your Health

What we are most interested in, of course, is the information about your health. In most doctors' offices, we find that the most efficient way to gather this information and to make sure we don't miss anything is through a health questionnaire. The questionnaire is usually one sheet of paper and asks questions about your current eye concern, your other medical conditions, your medications and drug allergies, and any surgery you've had in the past.

The questionnaire will also ask if any relatives have had medical problems because some medical conditions can run in families. We will also ask some specific questions about your general health. Finally, we ask some questions about your lifestyle – your occupation, and your alcohol, drug and tobacco use. These questions help us understand your visual needs as well as lifestyle issues that may affect your eyes and your health. If you don't know the answers to some of these questions, no worries. We have someone available in the office who can help you. We will review the questionnaire with you and help you with any of the answers that you may not know.

I hope that by knowing what will happen in a doctor's office you will be more comfortable and relaxed than I was on my way to the see the neurosurgeon about my neck. (It all turned out okay, by the way. He told me that I just needed to improve my posture, which I did, and in a week, all the pain that I'd had for five months disappeared, along with my fears of becoming Frankenstein.)

Let's now turn our attention to what happens during the eye exam itself.

11

THE
EYE EXAM

The first time I saw an eye through high-power magnification, its beauty enthralled me. I thought, how amazing it would be to spend my days examining the structures of this miraculous organ. Now, more than 25 years later, I still love this aspect of my work.

Here I'll explain to you what exactly is going on during an eye exam. If you've never had an eye exam, this chapter will tell you what to expect. But even if you've had many eye exams, you may have wondered what was going on with each step of the exam. Why was the technician asking me to move my eyes to the left or right? What was the doctor looking at with that light? Here I'll explain these mysteries.

An eye examination can be completed very quickly, but in those few minutes, a skilled eye-care team gathers a tremendous amount of information. Here are the things we do during a complete eye exam.

Visual Acuity

The first thing we check is your vision, or what we call your *visual acuity*. We want to know how well you can see. We discover your visual acuity by having you look at a chart of progressively smaller letters. The letters at the top of the eye chart are the largest letters and as you go down to the bottom of the chart, the letters get smaller. The smaller the letters you can see, the better your visual acuity. We may also check your near vision because the eyes may see clearly in the distance, but not at near, or vice versa. We check the visual acuity in each eye separately, so we know how well each eye is seeing.

We record your vision as a fraction. You probably know that "20/20" means perfect vision. Why do these numbers, expressed in this way, mean that your vision is perfect? If your vision is 20/20, it means that when you are twenty feet away from something, the normal eye could see that same thing just as well, also from twenty feet away. Your eye sees the same as a normal eye sees, so your visual acuity is perfect.

Now, if your visual acuity is 20/40, it means that when you are twenty feet away from something, a normal eye could see it just as well from forty feet away. You have to be twice as close to the object to see it as clearly as the normal eye sees it, so this is an indication that your vision is not perfect. And if your vision is 20/400, when you are twenty feet away from an object, the normal eye could see the same object just as clearly from 400 feet away. That's not very good vision. The lower the bottom number, the better the vision. Occasionally, I'll examine someone who has 20/15 vision. This person sees better than the normal person, because when they are twenty feet away from something, the normal person has to be fifteen feet away from it – that is closer to it – to see it just as well.

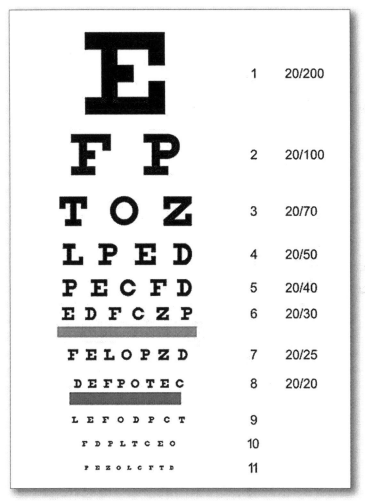

Figure 20: An eye chart to measure visual acuity

The Refraction

If your vision is not 20/20 or better, we have to discover the reason. There can be lots of causes for less than perfect vision, but the most common reason is that you may simply need glasses. All of the structures of your eye are working well, but the eye is just not able to focus the light properly. When an eye is not bending light rays properly, we say that it has a *refractive error*. We can help the eye bend the light and thus focus the light better by putting lenses in front of the eye. The process we go through to determine which combination of lenses is the best match for your eye is called *refraction*. In this process, we put a variety of lenses in front of your eye while you look at the eye chart, and we ask you to compare one lens to another and to let us know which lens helps you see clearer. By doing this, we can gradually find the lens that helps you see most clearly.

Sometimes we use loose lenses and hold them up one by one, but usually, it is easier if we use a *phoropter* – a gizmo that has all the lenses organized inside it. With a phoropter, we can just move a dial to give you the various lens choices.

We keep changing the lenses until we find the one that helps you to see the best. If for some reason the lenses do not improve your vision to perfect vision, then we know that there must be some problem other than a refractive error. In this case, during the rest of the eye exam, we try to discover what else is interfering with your vision.

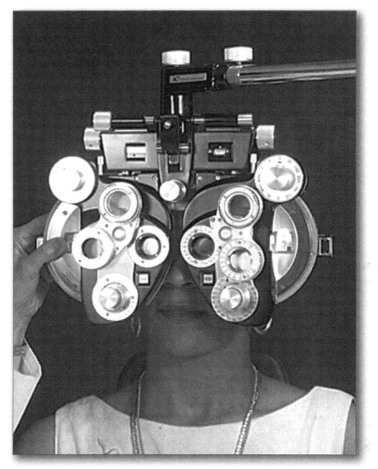

Figure 21: Phoropter. A phoropter is an organized collection of lenses that we place in front of your eyes to determine your refractive error.

Computerized Auto-Refraction

Sometimes, before performing the refraction, we will use a machine called a *computerized auto-refractor* to get a general idea of your refractive error. The auto-refractor doesn't really automatically do a refraction. It shines light rays into your eye and measures the way that those light rays bounce out of your eye. In this way it determines your refractive error. The auto-refractor gives us a good idea of your refractive error, but the measurements need to be checked and refined. For this reason, we can't really just write an eyeglass prescription based on auto-refractor results. But the measurements do help make the process of refraction much faster because they give us a starting point for the refraction that is often pretty close to your actual refractive error.

Peripheral Vision

In addition to your visual acuity, which measures your straight-ahead vision, we are also interested in your side or *peripheral* vision. We do a brief check of your peripheral vision by asking if you can see certain things in the periphery or edge of your vision. For example, the examiner may ask you to look straight ahead at her face while she holds up her fingers just outside your peripheral vision. As she brings her fingers into your view, she will ask you to tell her when you can see her fingers. Your peripheral vision allows you to see objects approaching from the side (like cars), and for this reason it is important for us to check it.

This check is not a precise test of your peripheral vision, but it is a good way to detect major problems. If we need more precise measurements of your peripheral vision, we can perform a formal computerized visual field test. In such a test, a specially designed machine flashes lights of various intensities in your peripheral vision, and each time you see the light, you press a button. In this way, we can map out the details of your peripheral vision. This formal visual field test is done most commonly with glaucoma and other types of optic nerve disease that damage peripheral vision. When we do these tests to check your peripheral vision, we say that we are checking your *peripheral visual field*. Your visual acuity is your straight-ahead vision, and your peripheral visual field is your side vision.

Color Vision and Stereo Vision

Besides visual acuity and visual field, there are other specialized forms of vision such as color vision and stereo vision. We don't routinely check color vision, but in special circumstances we may need to do so. In adults we also do not routinely check for depth perception, or what we call *stereopsis* or *stereo vision* – the ability to see objects in three dimensions. Since two eyes are needed to see in three dimensions, stereo vision testing is a measure of how well the eyes work together. In special circumstances, we may test your stereo vision.

External Exam, Pupils, and Motility

The external exam is an evaluation of the health of the structures surrounding your eyes. Are there any rashes or other skin problems on the face? Is an eyelid droopy? Is there symmetry of the facial structures? Are there lumps or bumps on the eyelids? These are the sorts of questions we ask when we look at these structures around your eyes.

The pupils are evaluated for their size, shape, symmetry, and their reactivity to light. During this part of the exam we shine a small flashlight into one eye, then the other, and then move the light back and forth between your eyes.

We also want to make sure your eyes are moving in coordination with one another. We ask you to look in various directions, or ask you to look at a small object as we cover and uncover each eye.

Intraocular Pressure

The eye, being a hollow ball, has a certain pressure inside it – the *intraocular pressure*. High intraocular pressure, even at levels that are not noticeable by you, can cause damage to your eyes. You can have high intraocular pressure for years and not even know it. One of the reasons we recommend routine eye exams is to detect high eye pressure before it causes damage.

We measure eye pressure in two ways: either with a puff of air; or with drops that numb the surface of the eye, with a glowing blue light, and an instrument that gently measures the pressure. The first method is called *non-contact tonometry*, the second, *applanation tonometry*. Different doctors' offices will use one or both of these techniques depending on the circumstances.

Slit Lamp Exam

A detailed examination of the front layers or *anterior segment* of the eyes is performed using an instrument called a *slit lamp*. The slit lamp is a microscope that is mounted on its side. It provides high magnification, letting us see the microscopic details of your eye. Typically, your doctor will examine the structures in order, from front to back.

During the slit lamp exam we first give careful attention to your eyelids and eyelashes, and then to your conjunctiva, the thin layer over the white part of your eye, which can become red during infection, allergies or irritation. Next we examine the tear layer that coats the surface of your eye. Deficiencies in the tear layer can cause dryness, irritation, burning and blurred vision. Beyond the tear layer is the cornea, and we use the slit lamp to examine its five layers: the corneal epithelium, Bowman's membrane, the corneal stroma, Descemet's membrane, and the corneal endothelium.

Right behind the cornea is the *anterior chamber* of the eye. This space contains a fluid called the *aqueous humor*. The fluid is usually clear, but in certain conditions it can contain blood, inflammatory cells, or proteins. With the magnification provided by the slit lamp, we can see the cells and proteins floating in this space, in the same way you would see dust or smoke floating in a beam of light in a movie theatre.

After checking the anterior chamber, we examine the iris, where we look for the neovascularization we discussed in Chapter 6. Right behind the iris is the lens. We can see a bit of the lens through the pupil, but to see more of it, we usually examine it again during the retinal exam, after the pupil

105

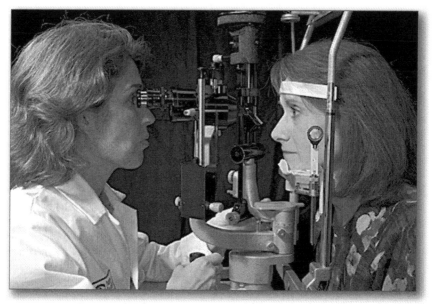

Figure 22: Slit lamp exam. The examiner is on the left, looking at the eye of the patient, who is seated on the right.

is dilated. With a dilated pupil we are able to fully examine your lens to see if a cataract is present.

The Retinal Exam

In order to get the best view of the lens and retina, we need to put drops into your eyes to open up your pupils and keep them open, or dilated. Usually, the pupil constricts when light shines into the eye. When we use our examining lights to look inside your eye, the pupil will constrict, making it very difficult for us to get a view of the structures behind the pupil. Without the pupil dilated, we can see only a portion of your lens and retina. Sometimes it is adequate to get this limited view of the retina, but usually, especially in diabetes, we need a detailed view of the entire retina. The only way to do this is to prevent the pupil from constricting. So we put special dilating drops onto the surface of your eye. The dilating drops open the pupil up, and prevent it from constricting when we use our lights to examine your retina.

Why is My Vision Blurry After the Drops?

The focusing ability of the lens allows us to see things that are near to us. The dilating drops temporarily relax this focusing ability of the lens and temporarily interfere with our ability to see near objects clearly. The distance vision is not normally affected by the drops. The dilated pupil also makes the eye sensitive to light. The dilating drops wear off in a few hours, and the vision returns to normal at that time.

It takes about thirty to forty-five minutes for the dilating drops to work, so you may be asked to spend some time in the reception area while your pupils are dilating. You will then go back into the doctor's office to complete the exam of retina and the lens – structures that cannot be fully examined through a small pupil.

To see the retina, we use special lenses, viewed through the slit lamp or through an instrument we wear on our heads called a *binocular indirect ophthalmoscope*. These lenses allow us to get a thorough three-dimensional view of the retina and related structures: the vitreous, optic disc, macula, the

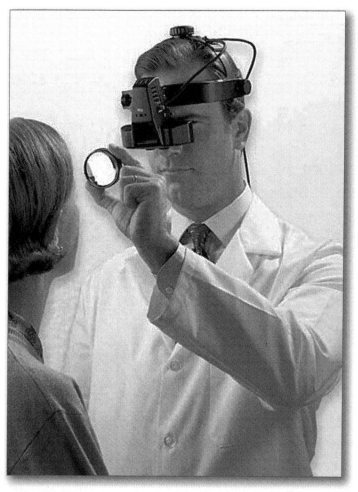

Figure 23: Binocular indirect ophthalmoscope. The doctor, on the right, uses the binocular indirect ophthalmoscope to get a three-dimensional view of the retina, including its far periphery.

retinal blood vessels, and the retinal periphery. This part of the exam may be a bit bright, but it usually lasts only a few minutes.

Who Does What in the Doctor's Office?

The complete eye exam as described above is a thorough medical evaluation of all the structures of your eye. As you can see, it is quite detailed. In the best offices, qualified eye-care technicians perform many of the tasks related to gathering information for the doctor. Typically, technicians perform the visual acuity and peripheral vision checks, the refraction, and the evaluation of the pupils, eye movements, and eye pressure. The doctor will perform the exam of the anterior segment with the slit lamp, and will perform the retinal exam with the various lenses and ophthalmoscopes, and analyze all this information to make the diagnosis and plan.

This then completes the eye exam. Using the information that we have gathered about your health and your symptoms, and combining it with the information that we have gathered from the examination of your eyes, we are then able to make a diagnosis. Based on the diagnosis, we then make a plan for treatment.

As a diabetic you should have a complete eye exam at least once a year. As you know, it is your retina that can be most severely affected by diabetes, and it is important that we examine it in detail at regular intervals so that we can monitor any changes.

12

SPECIAL
TESTS

D uring your visit to your doctor's office, there are a variety of special tests that we may perform to better understand your diabetic eye disease and to help guide decisions about your treatment. In this chapter I'll go over six of the most common tests we perform that are not part of the routine eye exam.

Retinal Photography

One of the most helpful special tests that we perform is retinal photography. We use a special camera that is designed to take pictures of your retina. You'll recall that the retina is the thin layer of nerves and blood vessels that coats the inside of the eye, and that it is the structure most affected by diabetic eye disease. Taking retinal photos helps us track changes in disease over time. Before the days of retinal photography, we would go to great lengths to precisely describe or draw what we saw in the retina. But a photo can capture the information instantaneously and more accurately. By comparing the appearance of your retina to previous photographs, we can determine whether your retinopathy is getting better or worse. Retinal photographs also help us document your response to treatment.

Now that digital retinal photography is available, the images can be viewed immediately. Even though retinal photography plays an important role in helping us monitor your retinopathy, often its most important role is to allow us to show you the changes inside your eyes. I really enjoy showing retinal photographs because it allows you to see exactly what I'm seeing, and for you to gain a deep understanding

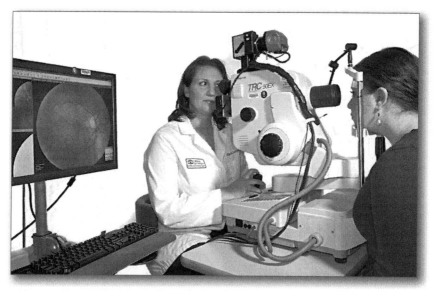

Figure 24: Retinal camera. The photographer, on the left, uses the retinal camera to capture a digital image of the patient's retina.

of your disease by seeing your own retina. This understanding helps you become a partner in battling the disease. You can see how close the swelling is to the macula, where the new blood vessels are growing, and how much bleeding or leaking is present. If you have any diabetic retinopathy, retinal photographs will become a regular part of your care. You have already seen lots of retinal photographs in this book.

Ocular Coherence Tomography

Ocular coherence tomography, or *OCT* (pronounced *oh-see-tee*), is a technology that became available in 2003. It has revolutionized the evaluation and treatment of retinal disease. OCT provides images of the layers of the retina, in the same way that a CT scan can look at very specific slices of the body. But instead of using radiation, like a CT scan, OCT uses light rays to create images of the layers of the retina.

To understand what OCT is doing, think of the retina as a cherry pie. Retinal photos capture an image of the surface of the pie. OCT takes a slice of the pie, and holds it up so that we can look at the layers – the thickness of the crust, the size and arrangement of the cherries, and the liquid filling.

In diabetic retinopathy, we use OCT to look carefully at the layers of the macula. It allows us to measure the thickening very precisely. So instead of saying there is "a little" thickening or "a lot" of thickening, OCT allows us to say that the central macular thickness measures 297 microns, or 452 microns, or whatever we measure. We can also look at images of the slices of the macula and see what type of

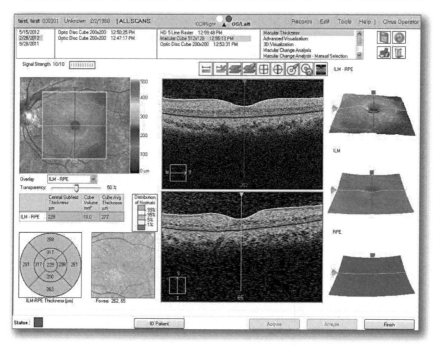

Figure 25: Normal OCT. This printout of a normal OCT scan combines several images. The image in the upper left shows the disc, blood vessels, and within the square, the macular area. The lower left image shows thickness measurements in various zones around the center of the macula. The images in the middle show two slices through the macula. The dip is the fovea, which is normally the thinnest part of the macula. The three images on the right show three-dimensional views of three separate layers in the macular area. You can see the amazing detail this OCT technology gives us, and how it can help us more accurately measure retinal thickness and see abnormalities.

swelling is present – is it diffusely swollen, or is the swelling in pockets? Which layers are affected the most by the swelling? In this way, OCT helps guide decisions about the

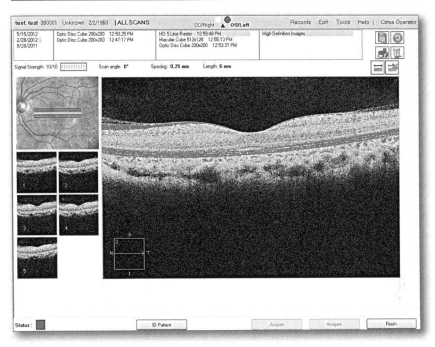

Figure 26: A high definition OCT scan through the macula, providing a higher resolution view of the layers of the retina.

specific type of treatment needed and the location of the treatment.

If you have macular edema, you can expect to have OCT performed periodically to measure the improvement or worsening of the macular edema and its response to treatment. With the most successful treatment methods, we use OCT every month to guide our decision-making process.

OCT technology continues to evolve. It is one of the most significant technological advances in ophthalmology. OCT has revolutionized our approach to many retinal diseases, and allows us to see layers of the retina in a way that was impossible before.

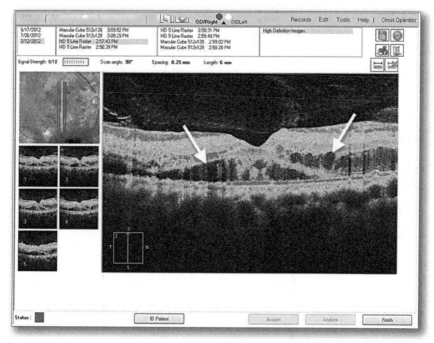

Figure 27: Macular edema. Compare the normal OCT in figure 26, to this OCT showing lots of dark areas (arrows) representing edema within the layers of the macula. The dip in the fovea is still present, but it is elevated by the swelling within the layers of the retina beneath it.

Fluorescein Angiography

Retinal photographs and OCT give us useful information about the appearance and structure of the retina. Photographs document the extent of disease and help us monitor changes in the appearance of the retina. OCT peers below the surface of the retina, into its deep layers and shows us areas of swelling or other structural changes that we cannot see on an examination or with retinal photography. OCT measures those changes very precisely.

Yet, as you may remember, the majority of damage that occurs from diabetes is related to the lack of oxygen in the retina, which is due to poor blood flow through the retina. Poor blood flow and poor oxygen delivery can result in loss of blood vessels, leaking blood vessels, swelling, and growth of new blood vessels. So, being able to evaluate blood flow through the retina would be extremely useful.

From the 1960's until 2015, the primary way to evaluate blood flow through the retina was through *fluorescein angiography*. With this test, a special dye called fluorescein is injected into a vein in the arm. As fluorescein travels through the blood vessels of the retina, we take a series of photographs. During the first minute of the test, photographs are taken every few seconds to capture the movement of the dye on its first pass through the retina. This first minute provides us with much of the critical information about the retinal blood flow. However, because we cannot photograph both eyes at the same time, we have to choose a "priority" eye whose blood flow will be evaluated during this first minute. If we want to evaluate the blood flow through both eyes, then we need to perform another fluorescein angiogram, usually on another day. After the first minute, we take further photographs over a period of 10-30 minutes.

Fluorescein angiography has been very helpful in evaluating areas of poor retinal blood flow. It also highlights areas of neovascularization that may not be visible on an exam. And because it shows leakage of dye from damaged blood vessels, fluorescein angiography can pinpoint the

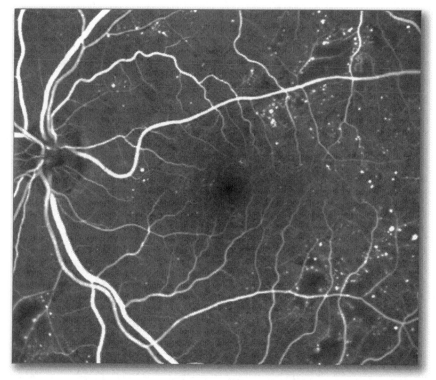

Figure 28: A fluorescein angiogram of the left eye. The many white dots are microaneurysms, most of which would not be visible on a photograph.

source of macular edema which can guide laser treatment. Fluorescein angiography has been a critical tool in evaluating retinal blood flow in diabetic retinopathy. However, a new technology has emerged which allows us to evaluate retinal blood flow without injecting a dye. Let's take a look at it now.

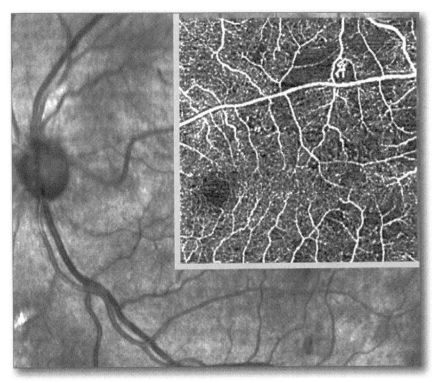

Figure 29: OCT-A. This is an OCT-A image of the same eye as in figure 28. The OCT-A image is limited to the upper right box in this image. While it does not show the microaneurysms as clearly as in the fluorescein angiogram, the small retinal blood vessels are more clearly visible in the OCT-A. In both the fluorescein angiogram and the OCT-A, loss of blood flow shows up as dark areas.

Ocular Coherence Tomography-Angiography

By 2015, advances in the resolution of OCT images, and advances in software led to the development of OCT machines that, in addition to viewing the layers of the retina, could also evaluate blood flow through the retinal blood vessels. This new capability is known as *ocular coherence tomography-angiography*, or OCT-A. The way OCT-A works is to take a bunch of retinal scans very quickly, and to then compare those scans to one another, and thereby construct a map of the blood flow. Not every OCT machine is equipped to perform OCT-A, so we need a special OCT machine to do this.

OCT-A has some advantages over fluorescein angiography. First, it does not require injection of dye, so this eliminates the risk and discomfort associated with the injection. Second, because the movement of a dye is not being evaluated, we don't have to choose a priority eye. Both eyes can be evaluated in the same sitting. Third, the images can be acquired very quickly, in a matter of seconds instead of many minutes, so the test is faster and easier than fluorescein angiography. Because there is no significant discomfort, risk, or inconvenience, OCT-A can be done regularly to evaluate retinal blood flow on an ongoing basis.

In diabetic retinopathy, OCT-A is most useful to evaluate blood flow through the macula. If you are not seeing well, but there is no macular edema present, we would like to know if the poor vision is due to poor blood flow. OCT-A can evaluate blood flow through the capillaries of the macula. If we find that the macular blood vessels are not carrying blood, then we know that macular ischemia is the cause of the poor vision. OCT-A has largely replaced fluorescein angiography as the primary test for evaluating macular ischemia.

Although OCT-A has significant advantages over fluorescein angiography, it does have a few limitations, and so certain situations remain where fluorescein angiography is more useful. One limitation compared to fluorescein angiography is that OCT-A cannot identify leaking blood vessels. So if there is swelling in an area of the retina, OCT-A cannot identify which blood vessels are leaking. In such cases, fluorescein angiography remains useful. Both tests can identify neovascularization, however, fluorescein angiography can also show leaking from NVD and NVE, which OCT-A cannot do. And because fluorescein angiography is capable of viewing more of the retina than a typical OCT-A, fluorescein angiography is still used to evaluate areas of widespread ischemia away from the macula or to find areas of neovascularization that are not visible on exam or OCT-A.

Fluorescein angiography and OCT-A are both important tests for evaluation of retinal blood flow in diabetic retinopathy. As the capabilities of OCT-A continue to advance, fluorescein angiography will be used much less often. Yet there remain some situations where fluorescein angiography adds to our understanding of blood flow through the retina.

B-Scan Ultrasound

One of the oldest technologies in medicine is ultrasound. Like x-rays, ultrasound is a way to look inside the body. But unlike x-ray, it does not use radiation; it uses sound waves. A gel is placed on the eye or the eyelid, and the ultrasound probe is placed on the gel. The probe sends out sound waves that bounce off of the structures inside the eye, and when those sound waves return to the probe, an image is formed.

Probably the most common use of ultrasound in medicine is during pregnancy. Ultrasound is used to look inside the mother's womb and evaluate the health of the baby, or to see if the baby is a boy or a girl. In the eye, most of the time we

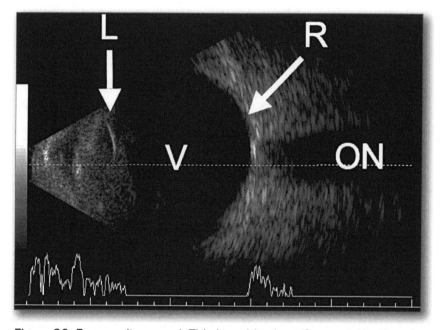

Figure 30: B-scan ultrasound. This is a side view of an eye that is looking toward the left. The ultrasound beam is traveling from left to right. The white curve on the left marks the back of the lens inside the eye (L). The ultrasound then passes through the vitreous cavity (V), and strikes the retina (R). You can see the back curve of the eyeball. Along the dotted line, behind the retinal curve, is the shadow cast by the optic nerve (ON). When a dense cataract, or vitreous hemorrhage blocks our view of the back of the eye, ultrasound images help us "see" into the eye to find out if the structures are in their normal position.

can just look directly at the retina. But in some cases, we might not be able to see inside the eye because something is interfering with our view. Maybe the cornea has become cloudy, or a dense cataract interferes with our view.

In diabetes, new blood vessels inside the eye can break and bleed, resulting in a vitreous hemorrhage. In some cases, there may be only a little bit of hemorrhage in the vitreous, and we may still be able to see the retina around the vitreous hemorrhage. But in other cases, there may be so much blood, or the hemorrhage may be so dense, that we cannot see the retina at all. In such cases we wonder, is the bleeding caused by the diabetic eye disease? Might it be from something else? Is there a retinal detachment behind the blood? Is there a tumor growing inside the eye causing the bleeding? Although it is very rare that the bleeding is caused by something other than diabetic retinopathy, we do not want to miss these other problems, and ultrasound helps us evaluate the structure of the retina when our direct view of the retina is blocked by vitreous hemorrhage or other problems.

Extended Ophthalmoscopy

Although you may not experience this as a separate test, when you look at a list of tests or procedures performed during your visit, you may see that a procedure called extended ophthalmoscopy was performed. Ophthalmoscopy is the part of the eye exam where we look at the retina. In people with significant retinal disease, like diabetic retinopathy, we spend extra time looking at the details of the disease, evaluating them, and documenting them, usually with a drawing. It is a more extensive retinal exam, and we call this extended ophthalmoscopy. If you have diabetic retinopathy, extended ophthalmoscopy will be performed regularly.

There are other tests that may be performed in special circumstances, but these six – retinal photography, OCT, fluorescein angiography, OCT-A, ultrasound and extended ophthalmoscopy — are the ones performed most commonly in cases of diabetic retinopathy. If you have diabetic retinopathy you can expect that at some point you will need one or more of these special tests, and likely on a regular basis.

13

THE

FOLLOW-UP VISIT

Whenever you have an eye exam you will be given a date for your next appointment. As we've discussed, the key to preventing blindness from diabetes is first to get your eyes examined, and then to get the recommended treatment. Coming back for your follow-up visits is part of the recommended "treatment."

If There is No Retinopathy

At the time you are diagnosed with diabetes and get your first eye exam, it is possible that you won't have any diabetic retinopathy. This doesn't mean that you will never need an eye exam again. You will need an eye exam at least once a year, every year, because the longer you have diabetes the higher the risk of developing diabetic retinopathy. For this reason it remains important to continue with your diabetic eye exams and to keep all of your follow-up appointments. How do we decide when to see you next?

Blood Sugar and Blood Pressure Levels

If your diabetes is out of control, diabetic retinopathy can develop or progress quickly. If your blood sugar has been high, we may recommend a follow-up eye exam in three to six months, even if you don't have diabetic retinopathy yet. Furthermore, your risk of developing severe diabetic retinopathy is higher if you have high blood pressure, so in such cases, we will monitor your eyes more often.

Severity of Retinopathy or Treatment

In addition to the status of your diabetes and your blood pressure, we also use the severity of your eye disease to decide how soon to examine you again. In general, the worse your diabetic retinopathy, the more closely we need to watch you. If your diabetic retinopathy is mild, and your diabetes is well-controlled, exams every six to twelve months are fine. However, if your diabetic retinopathy is more severe, or has shown significant worsening since your last exam, more frequent exams may be required. These may be needed as often as every one to three months.

You may also need to be examined more frequently after you've received treatment. For example, with the newer treatments (which I discuss in Chapters 18 and 19), monthly exams are needed.

Maria's Story

Returning for your follow-up exam is a vital step toward keeping your vision. It allows us to monitor your status and to catch problems early. I often tell the story of one of my patients, "Maria," who had very mild diabetic retinopathy for many years. She came in to see me every single year. But eventually she decided that because things were going so well, she could skip a few visits. Despite our calls and reminders, she did not come in for three years.

When she finally did return, it was because she woke up one morning with loss of vision in her right eye. During those three years that she had skipped her appointments, her diabetic retinopathy had quietly gotten much worse. It had become very severe. She had developed growth of new blood vessels. That morning, the blood vessels had ruptured, filling her vitreous with blood, resulting in loss of her vision. I was still able to help her, and her vision improved, but she needed many procedures, and her vision, even though it improved, never returned to normal.

Maria's chances for full visual recovery would have been much better if she had kept her follow-up appointments (even when everything seemed okay to her). If she had kept her appointments, we could have offered treatment before the disease was so severe, and we could have improved her chances of keeping her vision.

Be diligent about keeping your follow-up appointments. It is one of the best ways to beat diabetic eye disease.

PART III

TREATMENT

So far, you have learned how diabetes causes damage to your eyes, particularly to the retina. You have learned about macular edema, macular ischemia, and proliferative diabetic retinopathy. You have learned that these can all lead to severe visual loss. Additionally, you have learned about other eye problems that can be caused by diabetes such as cataracts, fluctuating vision, and double vision.

Furthermore, you have an understanding of what kinds of things you'll need to take with you to your eye appointment, and what happens during the eye exam. You have also learned the importance of the follow-up visit.

Through all of this, I have emphasized that diabetic eye disease can cause loss of vision. But just because vision loss *can* happen doesn't mean that it *has* to happen. Much of it is up to you. You now know that diabetes can be causing damage without you being aware that damage is occurring.

The key is to catch the problems early. And the only way to do this is by getting your eyes examined on a regular basis. I have taken people with all of these severe problems — macular edema, proliferative diabetic retinopathy, vitreous hemorrhage, tractional retinal detachment, and even neovascular glaucoma - and have saved their vision. It can be done. But the chances of keeping your vision are much better when the problems are found early. I've also seen many people with these same severe problems go completely blind.

If you haven't had an eye exam within the past 12 months, or if you have missed an appointment, I'd like you to put this book down and pick up the telephone and make an appointment for your eye exam.

Here, in the next few chapters I'll go over the main forms of treatment available for diabetic eye disease: laser, intraocular drugs, and surgery. In recent years there have been major shifts in the way we treat diabetic eye disease, and it has been an exciting time because the new treatments give better vision. Research is ongoing, and we expect that in the next few years we will have more weapons available to combat this blinding disease.

14

OPTOMETRISTS AND OPHTHALMOLOGISTS

Although both optometrists and ophthalmologists may diagnose diabetic retinopathy, for the most part only ophthalmologists treat diabetic retinopathy using lasers, medicine and surgery. The difference between optometrists and ophthalmologists can be confusing, as both are involved with diagnosing and treating eye disease, and both are called "doctor."

Optometrists attend optometry school, and have the letters "OD" after their name, which stands for "optometric doctor." Ophthalmologists attend medical school, and have the letters "MD" after their name, which stands for "medical doctor."

Optometrists provide optical care (through prescribing glasses and contact lenses) and medical care for common eye problems (through prescribing eye drops and oral medications). However, they do not typically treat diabetic eye disease with laser, injected medication, or surgery.

Ophthalmologists, on the other hand, perform all aspects of eye care – optical, medical, laser and surgical – with the full range of available medications and surgical techniques.

Optometrists and ophthalmologists work closely together in the diagnosis and treatment of diabetic retinopathy. But the treatments discussed in this section are performed by ophthalmologists.

15

LASER AND
MACULAR EDEMA

L aser is a major tool for the treatment of diabetic retinopathy, and was the first form of treatment that was
discovered. In the 1980's a large study of over 3,000
patients called the Early Treatment of Diabetic Retinopathy
Study (ETDRS) was done. It showed that people receiving laser for diabetic macular edema ended up with better vision,
compared to people who did not receive laser treatment. For
several decades, laser was the only tool we had to treat diabetic retinopathy, but beginning in 2005, new medications
that we inject into the eyes became available. Although these
new drugs have not completely replaced laser treatment, they
have decreased the need for laser, and I will discuss them in
Chapter 19.

What is Laser?

Laser is a type of light. Most sources of light send out light rays in many directions. Think of the light that comes from the sun, or from a light bulb. The rays of light are sent out in all directions, illuminating things all around them. A laser is different because it gathers and coordinates the light rays so that they all travel together in a single beam. Different types of lasers are capable of performing different tasks. When it comes to the human body, we use lasers for three main tasks: to heat tissue, to remove tissue, and to disrupt tissue.

We use all three types of lasers in eye care, but to treat diabetic retinopathy, we use lasers that heat retinal tissues. Lasers are used to treat both macular edema and proliferative diabetic retinopathy, but in different ways. Depending on the type of retinopathy, we treat different areas of the retina, and use different patterns of laser placement. In this chapter I'll discuss laser treatment for macular edema, and in the next, for proliferative diabetic retinopathy.

Macular Edema: Sealing Leaks

You'll recall that when the macula — the part of the retina responsible for your sharpest clearest vision — becomes swollen, we call it *macular edema*. Swelling occurs when blood vessels in the macula leak. The laser works to control diabetic macular edema by sealing up these leaks. As the leaks are sealed, the fluid has a chance to dry up, and the swelling decreases. As the swelling decreases, the vision loss may slow down or even stop. Sometimes the vision may even improve. What happens in your particular case depends on how bad the leakage is, how much damage has already taken place, and how well your diabetes and blood pressure are controlled.

Proof that Laser Works

It is important to have realistic expectations about the benefits of laser, and also about its limitations. For example, the ETDRS showed us that if 100 eyes have macular edema, and we watch these eyes for three years without treating them, at the end of the three years, about 25 of them will have significant loss of vision.

The ETDRS also showed us that if 100 eyes have macular edema, and we treat the macular edema with laser, at the end of three years, only twelve of them would have significant loss of vision. It's a simple comparison: no treatment results in 25% vision loss; laser treatment cuts the vision loss in half, taking it down to about 12%. Laser doubles your chances of keeping your vision longer.

What I point out to my patients is that even with the laser treatment, 12% of eyes will still have vision loss three years later. So the laser is not a magic wand that cures diabetic macular edema. Some eyes, even with laser treatment, continue to lose vision.

Goal of Macular Laser

The primary goal of laser treatment for macular edema is to slow down the damage. Over time, your vision may continue to get worse. The laser can help you keep your vision longer, maybe even forever. But in some cases the amount of leakage is overwhelming, or new leaks occur over time. In other cases the underlying high blood sugar keeps causing damage to the blood vessels, with ongoing leakage despite laser treatment.

I explain to my patients that using laser to fix the leaks in diabetic macular edema is a lot like trying to fix a leaking roof during a typhoon or hurricane. If you don't fix the leaks, the water will keep pouring in and can damage the inside of the house. Fixing the roof doesn't get rid of the damage inside the house, but it does slow down the leaking and slow down the damage. However, as long as the typhoon is blowing, more leaks can develop, causing more damage inside the house, and maybe even causing the areas that we had previously fixed to start leaking again. As long as your diabetes – your typhoon – is raging, the risk of ongoing damage and vision loss remains. If the vision gets worse after the laser, it's not the laser that's making it worse. It's the diabetes. It's not fixing the roof that causes the roof to blow away; it's the typhoon. This emphasizes the need to closely control the blood sugar and blood pressure.

But overall, we get better vision if we treat macular edema with laser than if we don't.

Macular Laser Patterns: Focal and Grid

When we treat a swollen macula with laser, we are trying to seal the areas that are leaking. Often, before we perform the laser, we do a few tests to help us to identify the exact location and extent of the leakage. These tests – the OCT and the fluorescein angiogram — help us to be more precise with the treatment. They also help us to monitor the response of your eye to the treatment.

We use various laser treatment patterns depending on the type of leakage that is present. If the tests show that the leakage is confined to a small area and we can pinpoint a specific leak, we place the laser treatment in that area. We call this "focal" treatment. However if the leakage is more diffuse — oozing from many different places — we may place the laser spots throughout the macula. We call this "grid" treatment. Sometimes the leakage may be a combination – a small localized area of leakage, and another larger area of ooze. In such cases we use a combination of focal treatment (to the small localized area of leakage) and grid treatment to the larger area of oozing. We customize the treatment to the particular conditions of your eye.

Although for decades, focal and grid treatments were the most powerful tools available for the treatment of diabetic macular edema, new drugs have changed that. In 2010 a study by the Diabetic Retinopathy Clinical Research (DRCR)

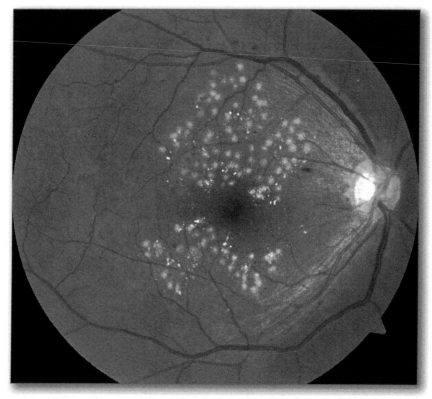

Figure 31: Macular laser treatment. The regular lighter areas are laser spots photographed immediately after laser treatment. Within the area of laser treatment, you can see smaller finer white areas that are hard exudates. Also visible are a few microaneurysms and retinal hemorrhages.

Network proved that a monthly injection of drugs is better than laser treatment for certain types of macular edema. Based on this research, the laser is no longer used as the primary treatment in people who have the appropriate type of macular edema. In such cases, we use medications, and use the laser if we need to. I'll discuss the details in Chapter 19.

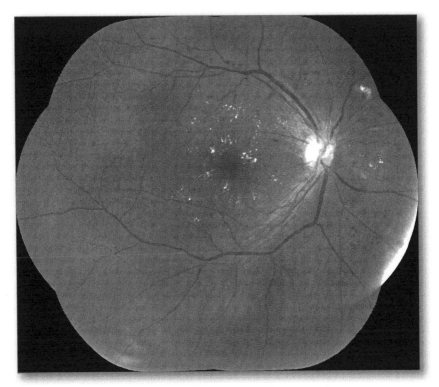

Figure 32: The same eye as pictured in Figure 31, immediately before macular laser treatment, showing the areas of hard exudates and microaneurysms that were associated with edema.

16

LASER AND PROLIFERATIVE DIABETIC RETINOPATHY

In proliferative diabetic retinopathy – the more severe form of retinopathy in which new blood vessels grow – laser has, for decades, been the most powerful tool for treating the retinopathy. And while in recent years, injections of drugs provide more rapid resolution of the neovascularization, laser remains a vital tool in the treatment of proliferative diabetic retinopathy.

"Pan-Retinal" Treatment Pattern

You'll recall that the new blood vessels that grow in proliferative diabetic retinopathy are dangerous because they can break and bleed, and also because they can cause traction and detachment of the retina. We need to get rid of these new abnormal blood vessels and we use the laser to accomplish this. However, instead of treating the macular area as we do for macular edema, in proliferative diabetic retinopathy we treat all the other areas of the retina. This form of treatment is called *pan-retinal laser*. Pan-retinal means "all over the retina." Of course, it's not truly "all over" because treatment does not include the macular area, but the treatment is much more extensive than for macular edema, and involves vast areas of the retina. Sometimes we call laser treatment, *photocoagulation*. So you may hear the phrase, *pan-retinal photocoagulation*, or *PRP* to refer to this pattern of treatment for proliferative diabetic retinopathy.

Proof that Laser Works for Proliferative Disease

We don't fully understand how pan-retinal photocoagulation works — how it makes the new abnormal blood vessels go away. But we know that it does, and that it reduces the risk of vision loss. How do we know this? Through a study that was performed in the years before the ETDRS, known as the Diabetic Retinopathy Study, or the DRS.

The DRS, which included over 1,700 patients, showed that treating proliferative diabetic retinopathy with PRP decreases the risk of severe visual loss. The study showed that if 100 eyes with proliferative diabetic retinopathy received no treatment, 50 of them experienced severe visual loss five years later. If 100 eyes received PRP, only 25 of them experienced severe visual loss.

Like the ETDRS, we found that treatment cut the risk of visual loss in half, and we found that it was also not a total cure. After all, 25% of eyes experienced severe visual loss even with treatment. Like in macular edema, laser for proliferative diabetic retinopathy can significantly improve your chances of keeping your vision, and keeping it longer.

Generally, I tell my patients with proliferative diabetic retinopathy that PRP can slow down the visual loss, or even stop it, and in many cases save the vision. But it's important to keep in mind that by the time an eye develops proliferative diabetic retinopathy, the eye is very sick and treatment becomes critical.

Why it Works

We do not understand exactly how PRP causes the new blood vessels to go away. One theory is that the laser destroys the areas of the retina that don't have sufficient oxygen. These areas produce a signal that causes the new blood vessels to grow. By eliminating these areas of unhealthy retina, we eliminate the signal, and the new blood vessels shrink away.

Another theory is that the laser, by removing the unhealthy retina, allows more oxygen to reach the healthier retina. Whatever the reason, pan-retinal photocoagulation does shrink the new blood vessels, and it is one of the major tools that we use to treat this severe form of diabetic retinopathy. It can save your vision.

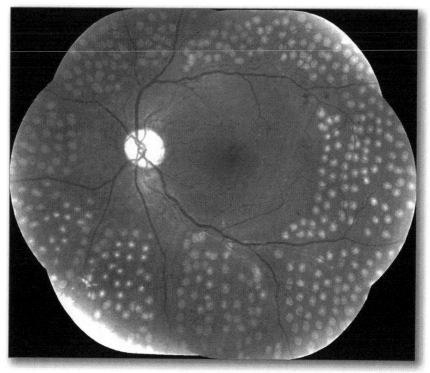

Figure 33: Pan-retinal photocoagulation, or PRP. Note that in contrast to macular treatment, the laser spots (the round white areas) are away from the macula. They extend much farther into the periphery of the retina than is visible in this photo.

17

WHAT'S IT LIKE TO HAVE LASER TREATMENT?

Although we often call it "laser surgery," laser treatment is not like a typical surgery. Because the laser is simply light, it can pass directly through the clear cornea and lens to reach the retina. For this reason, we don't have to make an incision of any kind to perform laser treatment.

Performed in the Office

You may remember that we can see the retina clearly because the cornea and the lens are clear and they serve as a window into the eye. The laser beam enters the eye through these structures. In fact, the laser is attached to the same instruments that we use to examine the retina: the slit lamp and the indirect ophthalmoscope. So it's something we usually do in the office, not in the operating room. You don't need to do anything special before or after the laser, and you can usually go on with your regular activities after the treatment.

The most common way to apply laser for diabetic retinopathy is through the slit lamp. Here is a picture of what laser treatment looks like. You can see that it's very similar to receiving an eye exam. The one difference is that we numb the surface of your eye with drops, and place a special lens on the eye to help deliver the laser beam.

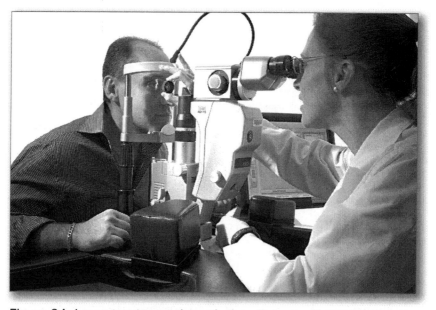

Figure 34: Laser treatment through the slit lamp. The ophthalmologist, on the right, holds a lens through which the laser beam is delivered to the patient's retina.

Macular Edema

For treatment of macular edema, you may need anywhere between about ten to two hundred laser spots. This depends on how much swelling there is and whether we are applying a few spots with focal treatment, or a more extensive grid treatment. Treatment for macular edema may take five or ten minutes to complete. During this time, you will see bright flashes of light as the laser is delivered, and you may hear a clicking sound from the laser as the shutter opens and closes to deliver the laser beam. The light can be bright, but as more laser spots are placed, your eye adjusts to the brightness.

Proliferative Diabetic Retinopathy

For proliferative diabetic retinopathy, because we have to treat a much more extensive area of the retina to get rid of the new abnormal blood vessels, the treatment is more extensive. It may require anywhere from 1,200-1,500 or so laser spots, and may take about fifteen to twenty minutes to complete. (Some lasers can apply the treatment much faster.) In more severe cases, we may need to place more laser spots – sometimes up to 3,000 or 4,000 or even more spots. In these cases, we divide the treatment into a few sessions spread out over several weeks.

Is There Pain?

Most people have no pain or discomfort at all during the laser treatment. Occasionally when we do pan-retinal photocoagulation we may encounter a sensitive area of the retina. If we know that you are experiencing discomfort, we will simply move away from that sensitive area and continue applying the laser. If you have continuous discomfort, we will give you some medicine to numb the deeper structures of the eye so that you're comfortable during treatment. It is rare to have any pain at all during laser treatment.

After the Treatment

After the laser treatment you are able to return to your regular activities. Your vision in the treated eye may be a little bit blurry from the dilating drops, and the world may look red as the eye adjusts back to normal lighting conditions during the few hours after the treatment.

Most people are a little bit apprehensive the first time that they get laser. This is understandable, but after their first treatment they realize how easy it is.

18

Injections and Diabetic Retinopathy: Dawn of a New Era

For decades, lasers had been our only tool in treating diabetic retinopathy. But in 2005 a new era dawned when Dr. Philip Rosenfeld, an ophthalmologist at the Bascom Palmer Eye Institute in Miami, took a drug that had been developed to treat colon cancer, and used it to treat new blood vessels growing inside the eye. The drug was Avastin, and Dr. Rosenfeld's injection of Avastin into a patient's eye revolutionized the treatment of many eye diseases, including diabetic retinopathy. If you have diabetic retinopathy, you will probably have a conversation about Avastin or similar drugs with your doctor. To understand these drugs and how they work, let's go back a few years to the 1990's.

Discovery of VEGF

During all the previous decades when we encountered new blood vessels growing inside patients' eyes, we suspected that there must be some sort of a signal — a chemical or a molecule — that was being made by the sick retina. We suspected that this signal was stimulating the growth of new blood vessels. If only we could discover that molecule.

Researchers spent years looking for the elusive molecule and in 1993, we found it. The molecule was named to describe its function: *vascular endothelial growth factor*, or *VEGF* (pronounced, *vej-ef*). It was a discovery that changed the way we treat many diseases in medicine. Its importance is hard to overestimate, and I believe that those who discovered it will one day receive a Nobel Prize. Here's why.

VEGF and Blindness

Worldwide, twelve million people are blind from macular degeneration and diabetic retinopathy. Growth of abnormal blood vessels in both diseases destroys vision. By finding the molecule that causes the growth of these new blood vessels, we found a target to attack. Attack VEGF, and new blood vessels can no longer grow. By successfully attacking this target, we can potentially prevent vision loss in millions of people. But the story of fighting VEGF did not begin with the eye. It began in a different part of the body.

Avastin is Born

In 2001 the innovative drug company, Genentech, received approval from the Food and Drug Administration (FDA) for a drug that could attack VEGF. We call this class of drugs *VEGF inhibitors* or *anti-VEGF drugs*. Genentech named the new drug Avastin (its chemical name is *bevacizumab*).

Avastin was developed and approved for the treatment of colon cancer. What does VEGF have to do with colon cancer? Well, as a cancer mass grows, it needs new blood vessels to bring oxygen to the cancer cells so that those cells can grow and spread. Avastin, when injected into the body, attacks the very thing that the cancer needs to survive, VEGF. By eliminating VEGF, the new blood vessels feeding the cancer stop growing. Without the new blood vessels and the oxygen they bring, the cancer mass shrinks or dies.

With the success of Avastin in treating colon cancer, Genentech turned its attention to developing an anti-VEGF drug specifically for use inside the eye. After all, VEGF was known to play a role in causing growth of new blood vessels in diseases such as macular degeneration and diabetic retinopathy. If a drug could be developed that could be used inside the eye, these diseases could be treated in a new way. The name of the drug that Genentech created is *Lucentis* (or *ranibizumab*), and molecularly it is a close relative of Avastin. After all, they both have the same function, which is to inhibit VEGF, so it makes sense that they would be similar molecules.

Dr. Rosenfeld's Insight

Dr. Rosenfeld was one of the researchers involved in testing this new eye drug, Lucentis. But while this research was going on, he began to wonder if Avastin, the colon-cancer drug that had already been approved, could be used inside the eye to eliminate the new blood vessels causing vision loss in macular degeneration. Although Avastin was not specifically approved for use inside the eye, any drug approved by the FDA for one disease may be used by doctors for other diseases, if there is a scientifically sound reason to do so, and if patients are informed of this *off-label* use of the drug.

One evening while driving home on the Rickenbacker Causeway, Dr. Rosenfeld had a revelation. He realized that Avastin, straight out of the bottle, would be safe to use inside the eye. This was important for two reasons. First, Lucentis was still being tested, and had not yet received FDA approval. So at that time, if you had macular degeneration you did not have access to any drug that could stop the new blood vessels from growing inside your eye, unless your doctor was one of the few in the country participating in the Lucentis studies. Avastin, on the other hand, had already been approved by the FDA. It was readily available throughout the country and could be used right away, as an off-label drug, by any ophthalmologist.

The second reason that this was an important insight has to do with cost. A single vial of Avastin could be divided into enough doses to provide treatment to fifteen or twenty eyes. The cost of Avastin per dose: about $60. Lucentis, on the other hand, when it eventually received approval, would cost $2,000 per dose. Dr. Rosenfeld's insight that Avastin was safe to use inside the eye gave ophthalmologists around the country immediate access to a low-cost way of treating macular degeneration and proliferative diabetic retinopathy.

The Shot Heard Round the World

Dr. Rosenfeld treated a few eyes with macular degeneration with Avastin and the results were remarkable. He presented the findings at the annual meeting of the American Society of Retina Specialists in Montreal in July 2005. It was the "shot heard round the world," starting a revolution in eye care. With Lucentis not yet approved, and therefore not available, ophthalmologists left the conference and immediately began using Avastin to treat patients. In the years that followed, studies were performed that showed Avastin and Lucentis have similar success rates. In situations where cost is an issue, Avastin continues to be favored by ophthalmologists and is the most commonly used drug to treat macular degeneration and diabetic retinopathy. Other VEGF inhibitors are available, and more are being developed by a variety of other companies.

VEGF Inhibitors and Diabetic Retinopathy

Although the initial ocular use of VEGF inhibitors was for macular degeneration, ophthalmologists soon began using them to treat diabetic eye disease, and with great success. If Avastin could get rid of new blood vessels growing in macular degeneration, then perhaps the same would hold true for proliferative diabetic retinopathy. And indeed, this turned out to be the case. For both of these diseases, the VEGF inhibitors worked like magic, causing the new blood vessels to just melt away, and in the case of macular degeneration, resulting in improved vision – something that was simply unheard of with treatments that existed at the time. A revolution in eye care had begun.

Furthermore, it was soon realized that VEGF inhibitors, particularly in diabetic retinopathy, not only cause new blood vessels to shrink away, but also seemed to decrease leakage from blood vessels. Thus, VEGF inhibitors could be used not only to treat proliferative diabetic retinopathy, but also macular edema, the most common cause of vision loss in diabetes.

But Are VEGF Inhibitors Better Than Laser?

Over the course of several years, we performed study after study, showing the usefulness of VEGF inhibitors in a variety of diseases involving retinal blood vessels. We were learning that VEGF inhibitors worked for both diabetic macular edema and proliferative diabetic retinopathy, but we had not yet compared their effectiveness to laser treatment. Sure, they worked, but did VEGF inhibitors work better, worse, or the same as laser?

In terms of diabetic macular edema, these studies culminated in 2010 with the publication of a landmark study by the Diabetic Retinopathy Clinic Research (DRCR) Network that showed that in diabetic macular edema, using a VEGF inhibitor gives better vision than treatment with laser alone. After decades of using laser alone, we now had a new weapon to fight diabetic retinopathy, and the new weapon was shown to be more effective than the old one. A major shift in the treatment of diabetic macular edema took place. Let's look a bit more carefully at the DRCR study and its implications.

19

VEGF Inhibitors and Macular Edema: The DRCR Network Study

The Diabetic Retinopathy Clinical Research (DRCR) Network is an innovative group of academic centers and private practices that work together conducting clinical research to improve the treatment of diabetic retinopathy. Our clinic has been one of the members of the DRCR Network, and I'll have to say, participating in the Network has been one of the most exciting aspects of my work. It has been an opportunity to be part of the leading edge of the treatment of diabetic eye disease. The DRCR Network is under the National Eye Institute, a branch of the National Institutes of Health.

The Network has performed many studies related to diabetic retinopathy. The study that proved the usefulness of VEGF inhibitors and their superiority over laser in some types of macular edema, is known as "Protocol I."

Whenever a new treatment comes along, we want to find out if it is better than the treatment we already use. So to answer this question a scientific study needs to compare the new treatment to the old treatment. The ETDRS and the DRS compared laser treatment (the new treatment at that time) to no treatment (which was the only other treatment option). Protocol I of the DRCR Network, which involved 850 patients, compared three new treatments to the old treatment (laser alone). Two of the new treatments involved giving VEGF inhibitors, and the third involved giving steroids. The most important outcome of this study was that the two groups of patients that received VEGF inhibitors ended up with better vision than those who received laser alone. The study showed that VEGF inhibitors worked, and that they worked better than laser alone. Let's take a more careful look at the results.

Measuring Visual Improvement

You'll recall that in the DRS and ETDRS, we looked at rates of visual loss. In the DRCR Network study, we looked instead at rates of visual improvement. How do we measure visual loss or visual improvement? Well, we use a special eye chart. You know from Chapter 11 that as you go down the eye chart, the lines get smaller. We talk about "lines" of visual improvement. So, for example, if someone can see 20/60 before treatment, and can see 20/30 after treatment, they have had three lines of visual improvement: from 20/60 to 20/50 is one line of improvement; from 20/50 to 20/40 is a second line of improvement; and from 20/40 to 20/30 is a third line of improvement. (This isn't exactly how it's done – we actually count "letters" of visual improvement, with five letters equaling a "line" — but in practical terms, it makes more sense to talk about "lines" of improvement rather than "letters" of improvement.)

Visual Improvement with VEGF Inhibitors

In the DRCR Network study, patients who received VEGF inhibitors showed more than two lines of improvement in their vision, whereas those who received laser alone had less than one line of improvement two years into the study. This is a remarkable difference. For the first time we were seeing that we could take people with diabetic macular edema and fairly consistently improve their vision. More patients who received the VEGF inhibitor (50%) had improved vision than those who received laser alone (30%).

Using OCT to Guide Treatment

At the time of the ETDRS, OCT technology did not yet exist, so we could not measure the thickness of the retina. Until the invention of OCT, the decision to treat was based purely on the clinical exam – on what the doctor saw when looking into the eye. If we saw thickening of the macula, and it met specific criteria, we would treat with laser. In contrast, Protocol I uses OCT technology to measure the macular thickness. This measurement, in combination with the clinical exam, is used to guide the decision to treat. If the OCT shows that the central macula is thick (more than 250 microns) and the vision is worse than 20/30 or so, we then initiate Protocol I.

Monthly Evaluation

Furthermore, one of the main differences between laser and VEGF inhibitors is that laser, by heating the tissues, causes a structural change in the retina that is more or less permanent. But it takes a while for the changes to take effect. For this reason, when using laser alone to treat diabetic macular edema, we usually wait three or four months before evaluating the eye again to see if more treatment is needed. Furthermore, once the structural changes from laser take place, the changes are there to stay, unless of course, more damage occurs from the diabetes, in which case more laser could be needed.

VEGF inhibitors, on the other hand, act quickly – in a matter of days – but their effects may not last forever. The drugs stay around in the eye for a month or so, and when they are gone, the problems can recur. So when we inject a VEGF inhibitor, it quickly mops up the VEGF that is present, but the sick retina is still producing VEGF. As the VEGF inhibitors wear off, the VEGF that is being produced by the sick retina builds up again, causing the problems to recur. To keep the problems controlled, more VEGF inhibitor needs to be given.

Since VEGF inhibitors last about a month inside the eye, we evaluate the effects of VEGF inhibitors on macular edema by using OCT on a monthly basis, and consider giving VEGF inhibitor as often as monthly.

New Treatment Strategy

Protocol I defined the treatment strategy that most of us are now using to treat diabetic macular edema. The basic strategy is that when diabetic macular edema causes the required thickening of the central macula (more than 250 microns) with a decrease in vision (worse than 20/30), we give four monthly injections of the VEGF inhibitor. Then using OCT measurements on a monthly basis, we determine whether or not more VEGF inhibitor should be given.

As long as improvement is occurring, we give more VEGF inhibitor. If the VEGF inhibitor is no longer improving the macular edema and there is still thickening, then laser may be added. The protocol is actually rather complex, but this is the basic idea behind it.

Fewer Lasers & Better Vision

Before the development of VEGF inhibitors, everyone with this type of macular edema would have been receiving laser treatment. When using VEGF inhibitors, the study showed that two years from the start of treatment, only 42% of patients needed laser. In other words, VEGF inhibitors alone controlled the macular edema in 58% of patients. Not only did the patients who received VEGF inhibitors need fewer laser treatments, their vision was better than those who had received only laser treatment.

Other Situations

Not all cases of macular edema fall within the treatment criteria set by Protocol I. For example, some patients may have macular edema that is less than the 250 micron threshold of Protocol I. But such a patient may fall within ETDRS criteria for treatment, and in such cases, laser alone may be the best treatment. In other cases, the vision may not be worse than 20/30 as set by Protocol I, but because the macula is thickened, it may again fall within ETDRS criteria for treatment, and again, the decision may be made to treat with laser alone.

But for the specific type of diabetic macular edema, where the center of the macula is thickened by more than 250 microns on OCT, and the vision is worse than 20/30, the first treatment is now VEGF inhibitors. Protocol I showed us that in this type of macular edema, the best vision comes with monthly visits, and OCT-guided treatment with VEFG inhibitors, supplemented with laser when needed. This means that if you have this type of macular edema, you need to visit your doctor more often; you need to receive treatment more frequently than with laser alone; and in the end this results in better vision.

Different Machines, Different Numbers

Different OCT machines have different methods of measuring the central macular thickness. The criteria for treatment used in DRCR Protocol I was based on measurements taken by the Stratus OCT machine. Newer machines use slightly different ways of measuring the central macular thickness, and so "normal" is generally higher than the 250 microns of the Stratus OCT.

For example, with the Cirrus OCT machine (made by the same company that made the Stratus), the central macular thickness needs to be more than 280 microns to meet Protocol I criteria for treatment. If we are using a machine other than the Stratus, we take the measurement techniques of each machine into consideration, and depending on the specific machine, we may use a threshold other than 250 microns to initiate treatment. So if your doctor recommends treatment at a number other than 250 microns, it is simply because of the OCT machine being used.

What About Steroids?

Besides comparing VEGF inhibitors to laser alone, Protocol I also evaluated another commonly used drug that is placed into the eye to treat macular edema: steroids. Steroids are potent anti-inflammatory drugs. Inflammation is thought to play a role in promoting leakage from the blood vessels of the macula. Therefore, steroids can decrease the amount of swelling in macular edema. There are several formulations of various steroids.

Before VEGF inhibitors were available, steroids were used in some cases of macular edema, with some success. However, the DRCR study showed that when compared to VEGF inhibitors, steroids have a higher risk of causing eye infection, raising eye pressure and forming cataracts. Furthermore, with steroids patients generally do not end up with better vision than with VEGF inhibitors. Nevertheless, sometimes we still use steroids, particularly in cases where the macular edema is resistant to VEGF inhibitors and laser. So although we don't use steroids routinely, in some circumstances we may discuss this option with you.

Other than the usual "out of the bottle" steroids, there are some innovative forms of steroids that have been developed for use inside the eye. Tiny pellets of steroids are injected into the eye. These pellets are designed to slowly release a steady dose of steroid to the macula over a period of several months or years. This avoids the need for ongoing injections. However, steroids can increase the risk of infection and of elevated eye pressure. For these reasons we usually prefer to use other treatments first, and if those fail, then we turn to steroids. Furthermore, because steroids can accelerate the formation of cataracts, we prefer to use them in people who will not be affected by this risk – namely, people who have already had their cataracts removed, or people who already have significant cataracts that will soon be removed.

And of course, because of the number of people affected worldwide by diabetic macular edema, new drugs are always being tested and developed, and in the coming years more options will likely become available.

Safety of Injections

In Chapter 7, I discussed cataract surgery and mentioned that any procedure around the eye (just like anything in life) carries some risk. Eye injections, especially with anti-VEGF drugs, are one of the most commonly performed office procedures in ophthalmology, with millions of injections being performed each year. Yet despite the fact that it's a relatively straightforward procedure – an injection performed in a doctor's office — there is a small, but real risk involved with each injection. The risk that we are most concerned about is the risk of developing *endophthalmitis* – an infection of the vitreous cavity that can lead to total destruction of the retina. The risk of endophthalmitis is small – less than 1/1,000 for each injection. But it's still there.

I tell my patients who need injections the same thing I tell patients when we discuss any procedure around the eye. I say, "I'm not telling you about the risks to make you nervous. I'm telling you about the risks because it's my responsibility as your doctor to make sure you know that, just like everything else in life, there are risks involved. Getting in a car has risks, walking down the stairs has risks, and an eye injection also has risks. The risks are small, but they're there. We do everything possible to decrease the risks, but we can't make the risks 'zero'."

The odds are in your favor, and getting the medications can significantly help your vision. Be informed, and make

decisions with your doctor based on sound information. But
don't let the risks overwhelm you. If you need treatment, the
risk of blindness from diabetes is much higher than the risk
of receiving treatment.

Does the Injection Hurt?

Most of the time when I tell my patients about VEGF inhibitors, and I tell them that I need to inject the drug into their
eye, they get scared. That's normal. People are afraid the injection will hurt. But you may be surprised to know that after
I complete the injection, most of my patients can't believe that
I've already given them the injection. That's because before
the injection we numb the eye. We use eye drops and other
anesthetics so you don't feel the injection. The anesthetics may
sting a bit, but the stinging goes away quickly and then most
people find that the injection has little discomfort – certainly
not as much as you would expect.

We have found that because of fear and nervousness, most
people find the first injection to be the most uncomfortable,
but after that first one, they know what to expect, and they
go on to get future injections without any hesitation. You'll
probably find that the injection, though it sounds scary at
first, can have very little discomfort.

20

VEGF INHIBITORS AND PROLIFERATIVE DIABETIC RETINOPATHY

Now that we've seen that VEGF inhibitors are better than laser to treat certain types of macular edema, it is reasonable to ask whether or not VEGF inhibitors also work better than laser for proliferative diabetic retinopathy.

You see, soon after Dr. Rosenfeld showed that Avastin could get rid of new blood vessels in macular degeneration, other doctors reported that it could also get rid of the new blood vessels in proliferative diabetic retinopathy. But the question remained, were VEGF inhibitors better for proliferative diabetic retinopathy than our standard treatment, pan-retinal photocoagulation?

In 2012, the DRCR Network launched a study, Protocol S, to determine how VEGF inhibitors compare to pan-retinal photocoagulation. The study, which included 304 patients, showed that patients with proliferative diabetic retinopathy who were treated with VEGF inhibitors had better visual outcomes than patients who received the standard laser treatment. Patients who received anti-VEGF treatment gained one more line of vision compared to those receiving laser treatment. Not only did treatment with VEGF inhibitors give better visual results, but patients who received VEGF inhibitors also experienced fewer vitrectomies, vitreous hemorrhages, and retinal detachments than those who received pan-retinal photocoagulation. They also had less peripheral visual field loss.

Proliferative Diabetic Retinopathy Alone

Does this mean that every patient with proliferative diabetic retinopathy alone (that is, with NVD or NVE only, and no macular edema) is now treated with VEGF inhibitors instead of laser? No, because as you know, anti-VEGF injections need to be given on an ongoing basis. Protocol S had good visual results because the patients had to get injections every four weeks. So, in order to consider anti-VEGF therapy as your only treatment, your doctor must be assured that you will return for more injections and follow-up visits. Consider, for example, that you only receive one injection and don't return for your next few injections, and as a result end up with severe progression of your proliferative diabetic retinopathy. In such circumstances it would have been better if you had received laser, than to have gotten the one injection and no further treatment.

While pan-retinal laser does cause some loss of peripheral and night vision, injections also have risks. With any injection into the eye, there is a very small risk of causing an infection inside the eye, which can lead to loss of vision. While this is exceedingly rare, it is a risk that does not exist with laser, and as always, we compare the risks and benefits of each option.

Cost and convenience can also be an issue with VEGF inhibitors. Typically, in the long run, the cost of ongoing repeat VEGF injections is more than the cost of laser treatment, and it can be inconvenient to visit the doctor's office every month.

So, if you have proliferative diabetic retinopathy without macular edema or other complications, your doctor will discuss these issues with you. Knowing that the better visual results of VEGF inhibitors require frequent ongoing injections which carry some risk not present with laser treatment, you and your doctor may decided that laser is the better option for you.

Proliferative Diabetic Retinopathy with Macular Edema

In those situations where proliferative diabetic retinopathy and macular edema are present together, VEGF inhibitors typically are used as first-line treatment. After all, Protocol I recommends that the macular edema be treated with VEGF inhibitors, and Protocol S supports the use for VEGF inhibitors for the proliferative diabetic retinopathy. So treatment with VEGF inhibitor helps both the macular edema and the PDR. Furthermore, because the method of laser treatment used in proliferative diabetic retinopathy can make macular edema worse, it is even more compelling to use VEGF inhibitors first, instead of laser, when PDR and macular edema are present together. In such cases, many of us start with VEGF inhibitors to quiet things down, and then if needed, add pan-retinal photocoagulation later.

Neovascularization of the Iris

VEGF inhibitors are clearly helpful when neovascularization of the iris (NVI) is present. You'll recall that once new blood vessels start growing on the iris, the situation is critical because these blood vessels can result in closure of the internal drainage system of the eye, causing the eye pressure to skyrocket. This can cause the vision to be permanently lost in a matter of days.

Pan-retinal laser was the main treatment for NVI, but it took time – often weeks – for the laser to cause regression of the NVI. So VEGF inhibitors, because of their rapid action, are now the first-line treatment for NVI. With VEGF inhibitors, abnormal blood vessels can melt away in a matter of hours, saving the vision. We then often follow this with placement of laser, which has a more lasting effect than the VEGF inhibitors.

I have several patients with severe NVI, who although they have received the full laser treatment, continue to develop new blood vessels on the iris. I give them Avastin on a monthly basis, and this keeps their NVI controlled. When we miss a month, the blood vessels grow back again on the iris, and the eye pressure rises. If you are unfortunate enough to develop NVI, you can be thankful that VEGF inhibitors now exist, because, used together with laser, they can save your vision.

Vitreous Hemorrhage

You'll recall that sometimes the new abnormal blood vessels that are growing on the retina can break and bleed, resulting in vitreous hemorrhage. Sometimes the vitreous hemorrhage is mild or localized; but sometimes it can be severe and diffuse, extending throughout the vitreous, and causing poor vision.

Traditionally we used laser to treat the neovascularization, as recommended by the DRS. However, when the vitreous was full of blood, the laser beam could not reach the retina. In such cases, we would wait for the blood to clear. As it cleared and the retina became visible, we would begin applying laser. If the blood did not clear after a few weeks, then we would remove it with surgery—a procedure called pars plana vitrectomy (which is the subject of the next chapter).

When we began to see that VEGF inhibitors could cause neovascularization to go away, we began to wonder if VEGF inhibitors could be of benefit in cases of vitreous hemorrhage. Maybe by closing down the new abnormal blood vessels, which are the source of the vitreous hemorrhage, VEGF inhibitors could speed up the resolution of the vitreous hemorrhage, or eliminate the need for surgical removal of the blood.

The DRCR Network Protocol N, which studied 261 eyes, showed us that VEGF inhibitors don't really help us avoid the need to surgically remove the blood. However, the study did show that using VEGF inhibitors in cases of vitreous hemorrhage does improve vision faster, does allow us to place more laser sooner, and does result in fewer re-bleeds.

As you recall, Protocol S showed that VEGF inhibitors can give better visual results than laser in proliferative diabetic retinopathy. While Protocol S did not specifically address cases of proliferative diabetic retinopathy that also have vitreous hemorrhage, the fact that it showed that VEGF inhibitors can be beneficial in proliferative diabetic retinopathy supports their general use. So when a vitreous hemorrhage occurs, and we don't have the option to consider laser immediately, both Protocol N and Protocol S support the use of VEGF inhibitors, and we use them routinely in cases of diabetic vitreous hemorrhage.

Before Surgery

There are two common situations when we use VEGF inhibitors for diabetic retinopathy a week or so before eye surgery. If proliferative diabetic retinopathy is present, and we need to perform a pars plana vitrectomy because of tractional retinal detachment or vitreous hemorrhage, we often give VEGF inhibitors before surgery to help close down the neovascularization, which consists of fragile blood vessels. It has been shown that giving VEGF inhibitors in these circumstances decreases the time of surgery, minimizes bleeding during surgery, and speeds up visual recovery after the surgery.

The second situation where VEGF inhibitors are used either before, during, or shortly after surgery is not related to proliferative diabetic retinopathy, but rather to macular edema.

We know that when we perform cataract surgery, the surgery can sometimes make diabetic retinopathy, particularly macular edema, worse. Some studies have reported that VEGF inhibitors, given in conjunction with cataract surgery, can decrease the risk of worsening retinopathy. Depending on the circumstances, we may recommend you receive a VEGF inhibitor around the time of your cataract surgery.

Individualizing Treatment

The approach to many of the situations that I have described is very individualized, and if you ask a room full of diabetic retinopathy experts how we would approach the treatment of a particular patient with diabetic retinopathy, you will get different answers. There are lots of ways to use VEGF inhibitors in combination with laser for treatment of retinal disease, and many approaches are reasonable and work well.

The DRCR Protocol I study lays out a fairly clear roadmap for the treatment of a specific form of diabetic macular edema. Protocol S shows us that it is reasonable to use anti-VEGF drugs for proliferative diabetic retinopathy. And Protocol N supports the use of VEGF inhibitors in vitreous hemorrhage. However, not every patient matches the situation of the patients in those studies. We do not have the results of large studies to answer every question. There will always be unique situations. In such cases, treatment plans which may combine VEGF inhibitors with laser need to be individualized, and you will participate in your treatment decisions with your doctor. As new knowledge becomes available, new approaches will evolve.

In the next chapter we will look at the most common surgery performed to treat severe forms of diabetic retinopathy, the pars plana vitrectomy.

21

Going to the Operating Room: The Pars Plana Vitrectomy

O nce in a while diabetic retinopathy can become so severe that treatment with lasers and injections is not enough. In some severe cases you need to go to the operating room for a surgical procedure. The surgical procedure that we perform most often for these severe complications of diabetic retinopathy is called the *pars plana vitrectomy*. The name of this procedure comes from the fact that we are removing vitreous (*vitrectomy*), through incisions made in a part of the eye called the *pars plana*, which is located through the sclera, a few millimeters from the edge of the cornea.

Vitreous Hemorrhage

There are two common reasons for a pars plana vitrectomy in diabetic eye disease. The first reason is to remove blood that has filled the inside of the eye. When new blood vessels grow inside the eye they can break and bleed. The blood can fill the large chamber known as the *vitreous chamber*. This kind of bleeding is called a vitreous hemorrhage.

Often a vitreous hemorrhage will go away with time. Your body can gradually absorb the blood. But in some cases, the blood does not go away, or does not go away as quickly as we had hoped, and so we remove it.

The pars plana vitrectomy is the procedure used to remove the vitreous, and the blood along with it. The vitreous that we remove is replaced naturally by clear fluid that your body produces. Because the blood has been removed, the light can get to get to the retina unimpeded, and vision can improve.

Tractional Retinal Detachment

A second reason for a pars plana vitrectomy in diabetic eye disease is to repair a tractional retinal detachment. Sometimes, the new blood vessels that grow on the retina can have fibrous elements associated with them. These fibrous elements can contract and pull on the surrounding retina. Sometimes they can cause so much traction on the retina that the retina tents up from its normal position. This is called a retinal detachment, because the retina has separated or detached from the underlying structures of the eye.

Because the detachment is caused by the contraction of these fibrous elements and by the traction they place on the retina, we call the detachment a tractional retinal detachment. Just as with retinal edema, a tractional retinal detachment is most significant when it affects the macula, the specialized area of the retina involved with your sharpest clearest vision. If there is traction on the macula, or if the macula detaches, your vision can get worse.

A pars plana vitrectomy for tractional retinal detachment can be a fairly complex operation. In addition to removing the vitreous from the eye, the traction caused by various fibrous membranes has to be released. Sometimes the membranes can be peeled from the surface of the retina, but often the membranes are integrated into the retina, making complete removal impossible. Our goal during this type of surgery is not necessarily to remove all the membranes and fibrous elements, but rather to release the traction and to flatten the retina. During the procedure we may use lasers to help tack down areas of the retina, and also to give adequate treatment to the underlying proliferative diabetic retinopathy that led to the tractional retinal detachment.

Other Reasons

There are two other, less common reasons for a pars plana vitrectomy in diabetes. The first is that in some types of macular edema, the macula is swollen because the vitreous (not

Gas and Oil

Sometimes the retina may need some additional help re-attaching, and staying attached. In these cases we may place a gas bubble inside the eye at the end of the surgery to help keep the retina in place. The gas bubble goes away by itself over a few days or weeks. During some of that time you may need to lie in a special position so that the gas bubble is exactly where it needs to be. Because gas expands at higher elevations, it is not safe to fly with a gas bubble in your eye.

Gas bubbles are the most common way to give the retina some extra help in reattaching. But sometimes we use another substance, silicone oil. The oil has the advantages of staying in place longer than gas, and does not require you to be positioned in any special way after the surgery. And because oil does not expand significantly, it is okay to fly with silicone oil in your eye. But it does have the disadvantage of usually needing to be removed some months later. Removing the oil requires another trip to the operating room.

a membrane) is tugging on the retina. This is called *vitreo-macular traction,* or VMT. Releasing the vitreous traction can improve the edema. However, in 2012 a new drug was approved that can relieve VMT in some people, and we may offer it to you as an option. The name of the drug is *ocriplasmin.*

The second uncommon reason for a pars plana vitrectomy is for a condition called *endophthalmitis*. This is an infection that develops in the vitreous chamber, as a result of bacteria being introduced into the eye, as can happen through an injection site. Pars plana vitrectomy in endophthalmitis is performed to remove the infected vitreous.

Realistic Expectations

In many cases your vision can improve significantly after pars plana vitrectomy. However, I tell my patients to keep in mind that the pars plana vitrectomy is needed because the eye is very sick. Because the eye has already had severe damage, the chance of full visual recovery may be limited. The chance of recovery depends on the state of the eye before surgery. If the eye has very little traction, it will have a better chance of good vision after pars plana vitrectomy. If there is extensive traction and retinal detachment, the chances of good vision may be limited. The doctor performing your surgery can advise you about the prognosis in your individual situation.

PART IV

CONTROLLING DIABETES
AND GETTING HEALTHY

I've spent the majority of this book talking about two of the things you can do to avoid blindness from diabetes: get your retina examined every year; and follow your doctor's advice diligently regarding treatment and follow-up. Basically, it is a plan to find problems and treat these problems. These two steps are key, and can make the difference between keeping your sight or going blind. But there is another step you can take that can have a huge impact on your vision: control your diabetes, and the conditions that often accompany and exacerbate diabetes - obesity, hypertension, high cholesterol and smoking.

Volumes have been written on each of these subjects. I mention the importance of each one briefly here. I encourage you to learn more about each of them. These five areas can affect your health as a diabetic more than anything else, and controlling them can have a tremendous impact on your health and your vision.

Diabetes Control

You already understand that high blood sugar causes damage to blood vessels, and those damaged blood vessels cannot adequately deliver oxygen to your organs. This poor blood flow and poor oxygen delivery lead to all of the complications we see in diabetes. So, controlling blood sugar is a major factor in controlling the damage that occurs from diabetes – not just to the eye, but also the feet, the sexual organs, the kidneys, the heart, and the brain. If you can control your blood sugar, then your risk of complications goes way down.

One important measure of glucose control is something called *hemoglobin A1c*. While your blood sugar measurements tell us how your blood sugar is doing at a particular moment in time, they really don't tell us what your blood sugar was like last week or last month. Hemoglobin A1c, on the other hand, tells us how well your blood glucose has been controlled over the past few months. We like to see hemoglobin A1c measurements below seven.

Obesity

Obesity is a major cause of diabetes, and controlling diabetes is closely connected to losing extra body fat. More than 90% of people with diabetes have obesity, and losing weight will go a long way toward controlling your blood sugar. There are many ways to do this, and other doctors have written extensively about it. I encourage you to learn more about the steps you can take to lose weight.

Blood Pressure

There is another factor that can exacerbate the damage from diabetes: high blood pressure. If the pressure inside the blood vessels is high, you can guess that the blood vessels themselves can get damaged. High blood pressure in the presence of diabetes is another blow to the blood vessels. Furthermore, in the case of the retina, when the blood vessels are leaking, high blood pressure can make the leaking worse. It's similar to when a water hose has a leak, and someone turns up the pressure inside the hose. The leak will get worse. So controlling high blood pressure can also decrease your risk of vision loss from diabetes, as well as your risk of stroke, heart attack, and other problems caused by damaged blood vessels.

Cholesterol and Fat

High cholesterol and fats are two other enemies of healthy blood vessels. High cholesterol contributes to blood vessel damage, and high fats can make your cholesterol levels worse. Extremely high fats can leak from the blood vessels and can thicken the blood, causing it to move slowly and deliver oxygen poorly.

Smoking

A fifth contributor to the complications of diabetes is smoking. Diabetes damages blood vessels, and smoking damages blood vessels. Either one by itself is bad, but together, they are a disaster. The most difficult cases of diabetic retinopathy that I deal with are in patients who cannot stop smoking. Smoking is an addiction, and like any addiction it can be extremely difficult to overcome, but it is possible. Your doctor can guide you to programs and medications that can make it easier to quit smoking.

Lifestyle: The Key to Health

Although it is beyond the scope of this book to discuss all of these problems in detail, it is extremely important for our increasingly unhealthy society to understand that we are all at risk for developing diabetes, and that in most cases, diabetes can be prevented, controlled and even reversed. The same holds true for other accompanying diseases like obesity, hypertension, high cholesterol, and smoking. Gaining an understanding of these five conditions is the ultimate key to understanding your health and preventing blindness from diabetes.

As you gain a deeper understanding of these diseases, you'll find that they are mostly "lifestyle" diseases. The way you live – the food you eat, how much you exercise, what you choose to inhale – influences your health more than almost anything else. You may be surprised to learn that some simple changes in your lifestyle can vastly improve your health, decrease your reliance on medication, and improve your chances of keeping your vision.

FINAL THOUGHTS

I hope you have enjoyed this book. As I mentioned in the introduction, I have done my best to take the most important information – the stuff you need to know in order to keep your vision and your independence, to calm your fears, and to give you peace of mind – and to share it with you in a clear and easy to understand way. I hope I have been successful.

You now have more knowledge about diabetic eye disease than most people in the world. Some of the greatest rewards come from helping others, so please share your knowledge with your friends and family, so that they too may start the journey to a lifetime of good vision.

Knowledge should lead to action, and the three actions that I have emphasized throughout this book are: get your eyes examined every year; get treatment when it's recommended; and control your diabetes. These three actions will guarantee that you'll keep the best vision you can have.

As you walk this path toward keeping your vision, be patient with yourself. As you've learned, the things you need to do are fairly simple. But just because something is simple, doesn't mean it's easy. Why? Because diabetes doesn't take a day off, and neither do the thousand other things that need your attention every day of your life. Sometimes you'll get too busy. Sometimes you'll forget. Sometimes you'll just be too tired to do what you need to do for your health. That's okay. But don't give up. Keep coming back to the things you've learned here. They'll remind you, boost your motivation, and get you back on track.

I wish you all the best on your journey. Thank you for spending this part of it with me.

GLOSSARY

A

Anti-VEGF drugs – see *VEGF inhibitors*

Avastin – a commonly used VEGF-inhibitor, used to treat many diseases of the eye including macular edema and neovascularization. Its chemical name is *bevacizumab*. It costs less than 10% of the other major VEGF inhibitor, Lucentis.

B

Background diabetic retinopathy – another way of saying *non-proliferative diabetic retinopathy*

Bevacizumab – see *Avastin*

C

Capillaries – the smallest blood vessels in the body, they form a network to supply blood and oxygen to cells and tissues

Cones – along with rods, cones are one of the two types of photoreceptors. Cones are responsible for color vision and daytime vision.

Cornea – the clear dome at the front of the eye, which covers the iris. The cornea is the first structure that light passes through as it enters the eye.

Cotton-wool spots – yellow-white areas of the superficial layer of the retina. They are the result of loss of blood flow from blocked blood vessels, and can be thought of as tiny "strokes" of the retina.

D

Diabetic retinopathy – damage of the retina caused by diabetes

Diabetic Retinopathy Clinical Research Network – a network of academic centers, community clinics and private practices working together to further knowledge about diabetic eye disease. The network is under the auspices of the National Institutes of Health and the National Eye Institute.

Diabetic Retinopathy Study – see *DRS*

Disc – see *optic disc*

Dot or blot hemorrhage – bleeding in the deeper layers of the retina

DRCR – abbreviation for *Diabetic Retinopathy Clinical Research Network*

DRS – abbreviation for *Diabetic Retinopathy Study*, an important study performed in the late 1970's that showed that people treated with laser for proliferative diabetic retinopathy ended up with better vision than those who received no laser treatment

E

Early Treatment of Diabetic Retinopathy Study – see *ETDRS*

Edema – an area of swelling

Endophthalmitis – an infection that develops in the vitreous chamber as a result of bacteria introduced into the eye. It is a vision-threatening emergency.

ETDRS – abbreviation for *Early Treatment of Diabetic Retinopathy Study*, an important study performed in the 1980's that showed that people treated with laser for macular edema ended up with better vision than those who received no laser treatment.

F

FDA – abbreviation for *Food and Drug Administration*, the US government agency charged with monitoring and approving new drugs that are being developed.

Fibrovascular changes – a combination of fibrous elements and blood vessels that results from changes in neovascular tissues, and which often leads to tractional retinal detachments

Flame hemorrhage – bleeding in the superficial layers of the retina

Floaters – opacities in the vitreous that cast a shadow on the retina and appear as objects floating and moving in your vision. These may be a natural part of aging, or can be a sign of vitreous hemorrhage.

Fovea – the very center of the macula, which is responsible for your sharpest clearest vision

G

Glucose – the main type of sugar in the blood. It is the major source of energy for the cells in your body. We often refer to it as "sugar," or "blood sugar."

H

Hard exudates – yellow glistening collections of fats and proteins that have leaked out of damaged retinal blood vessels into the retina

Hemorrhage – an area of bleeding

Hemorrhage, intra-retinal – bleeding within the retina. These areas of bleeding are one of the first findings of non-proliferative diabetic retinopathy.

Hemorrhage, preretinal – bleeding that is immediately in front of the retina, wedged between the surface of the retina and the vitreous. A pre-retinal hemorrhage is a sign of proliferative diabetic retinopathy.

Hemorrhage, retinal – another name for *intra-retinal hemorrhage*

Hemorrhage, vitreous - bleeding into the vitreous cavity. In diabetes, this most commonly occurs as a result of proliferative diabetic retinopathy, in which new abnormal blood vessels break and bleed.

I

Intra-retinal hemorrhage – see *hemorrhage, intra-retinal*

Iris – the colored blue or brown part of the eye. The iris can develop neovascularization, which is a sign of severe proliferative diabetic.

IRMA – abbreviation for *intra-retinal microvascular abnormality*, a hallmark, along with venous beading, of severe background diabetic retinopathy. It is marked by unusual changes in the tiny blood vessels within the retina. Most often, IRMA looks like unusual loops, or squiggly blood vessels.

Ischemia – loss of blood flow to an area, often resulting in loss of function. In the retina, small areas of ischemia are most often seen as cotton-wool spots.

L

Laser – abbreviation for *Light Amplified Stimulation of Emitted Radiation*. Lasers are a type of light beam that are used to treat diabetic retinopathy.

Lucentis – a commonly used VEGF-inhibitor, used to treat many diseases of the eye including macular edema and neovascularization. Its chemical name is *ranibizumab*. It costs about $2,000 per dose.

M

Macula – the darker area of the retina responsible for producing your sharpest clearest vision

Macular edema – swelling of the macula. This is the main cause of vision loss in diabetes.

Macular ischemia – loss of blood flow to the macula, often resulting in loss of vision

Microaneurysms – tiny bulges or out-pouchings of the small retinal blood vessels. Microaneurysms are one of the first signs of diabetic damage.

N

Neovascular glaucoma – elevated pressure inside the eye caused by growth of new blood vessels on the iris. It is extremely dangerous to the eye

Neovascularization – growth of new blood vessels. This is the hallmark of proliferative diabetic retinopathy.

Neovascularization elsewhere (NVE) – growth of new blood vessels in areas of the retina other than on the optic disc

Neovascularization of the disc (NVD) – growth of new blood vessels on the optic disc

Neovascularization of the iris (NVI) – growth of new blood vessels on the iris, which often leads to neovascular glaucoma

Non-proliferative diabetic retinopathy – one of the two main kinds of diabetic retinopathy. In non-proliferative diabetic retinopathy, there are no new blood vessels growing inside the eyes, but there are other signs of diabetic damage such as microaneurysms, cotton-wool spots, retinal hemorrhages, edema, venous beading and IRMA. Non-proliferative diabetic retinopathy is commonly called, *background diabetic retinopathy.*

NPDR – abbreviation for *non-proliferative diabetic retinopathy*

NVD – abbreviation for *neovascularization of the disc*

NVE – abbreviation for *neovascularization elsewhere*

NVI – abbreviation for *neovascularization of the iris*

O

Occipital lobes – the part of the brain, located at the back of the head, that is involved with turning the electrical signals sent from the eye into pictures that you can understand. It is the part of the brain involved in vision.

OCT – abbreviation for *ocular coherence tomorgraphy*

Ocriplasmin – a drug approved by the FDA in 2012 which can be used as an alternative to surgery to treat vitreomacular traction

Ocular coherence tomography – commonly abbreviated, *OCT*. A technology that allows us to see structural changes within the retinal layers, and to measure those changes very precisely. It is routinely used in evaluating and treating macular edema.

Off-label – use of a drug to treat a disease other than the one it was specifically approved by the FDA to treat. For example, Avastin was approved by the FDA to treat colon cancer, however it is also used to treat diabetic retinopathy, macular degeneration, and a variety of ocular inflammatory and vascular diseases. The use of Avastin to treat these eye diseases is "off-label" use. It is being used to treat diseases other than the one the FDA has "labelled" it for. Many drugs are used off-label.

Ophthalmologist – one of the two types of eye doctors. Ophthalmologists are medical doctors (MD) and are trained to provide all aspects of eye care: optical, medical, surgical and laser treatment. They work closely with optometrists.

Ophthalmoscope – an instrument that allows the doctor to look inside the eye and carefully examine the retina

Optic cup – the central excavated area of the optic nerve, which can become enlarged in glaucoma

Optic disc – the surface of the optic nerve, visible as a prominent round yellow/white area on the retinal surface

Optic nerve – the bundle of 1.2 million nerve fibers that transmits electrical signals from the eye to the brain

Optometrist – one of the two types of eye doctors. Optometrists are not medical doctors, but rather optometric doctors (OD). They are trained to provide optical and medical eye care, but do not typically perform surgery, laser, injections or other treatments for diabetic eye disease. They work closely with ophthalmologists.

P

PDR – abbreviation for *proliferative diabetic retinopathy*

Photocoagulation – the word used to refer to laser treatment of the retina

Photoreceptors – the specialized cells deep in the retina which convert light that comes into the eye, into electrical signals that go to the brain. There are two types of photoreceptors: rods and cones.

Pre-retinal hemorrhage – see *hemorrhage, preretinal*

Proliferative diabetic retinopathy – one of the two main kinds of diabetic retinopathy. In proliferative diabetic retinopathy, new blood vessels grow (or *proliferate*) in the eye.

PRP - abbreviation for *pan-retinal photocoagulation*, which is a pattern of laser treatment that is placed throughout much of the retina. The primary reason to use PRP is to treat proliferative diabetic retinopathy.

Pupil – the black hole in the center of the iris that controls the amount of light entering the back of the eye. When light becomes bright, the pupil gets smaller to let in less light; when light becomes dim, the pupil gets bigger to let in more light.

R

Ranibizumab – see *Lucentis*

Retina – the thin layer of nerves and blood vessels that coats the inside of the eyeball, and that is most sensitive to diabetic damage

Retinal hemorrhage – see *hemorrhage, retinal*

Retinopathy – damage or disease of the retina

Rods – along with cones, rods are one of the two types of photoreceptors. Rods are responsible for vision in dim light.

S

Sclera – the white part of the eye that you see when you look at your eye in a mirror. The sclera and the cornea together make up the wall of the eyeball.

Sugar – see *glucose*

T

Tractional retinal detachment – separation of the retina from its normal position as a result of membranes pulling the retina from its normal position. This may occur during proliferative diabetic retinopathy when fibrovascular membranes form, and can lead to vision loss

V

Vascular endothelial growth factor – a molecule that stimulates the growth of new blood vessels and can cause swelling of the macula. It is known most commonly by its abbreviation, *VEGF.*

Venous beading – a hallmark, along with IRMA, of severe background diabetic retinopathy. Veins become narrow in some areas, resembling a string of beads or sausages.

VEGF – abbreviation for *vascular endothelial growth factor*

VEGF inhibitors – drugs that interfere with the action of VEGF, thereby treating neovascularization and macular edema. The most commonly used VEGF inhibitors are Avastin (bevacizumab) and Lucentis (ranibizumab).

Vitreo-macular traction – traction on the macula caused by vitreous, which can lead to macular edema

Vitreous – the clear jelly that fills the vitreous chamber, the large cavity at the back of the eye

Vitreous floaters – see *floaters*

Vitreous hemorrhage – see *hemorrhage, vitreous*

PHOTO CREDITS

Figure 1: National Eye Institute, National Institutes of Health
Figure 2: Sarah Cartwright; Creative Commons: Attribution, Share-Alike
Figure 3: Wikispaces; Creative Commons: Attribution, Share-Alike
Figure 4: Marianas Eye Institute
Figure 5: Wikispaces; Creative Commons: Attribution, Share-Alike
Figure 6: Marianas Eye Institute
Figure 7: Marianas Eye Institute
Figure 8: The Community Eye Health Journal
Figure 9: Marianas Eye Institute
Figure 10: Marianas Eye Institute
Figure 11: RetinaGallery.com
Figure 12: RetinaGallery.com
Figure 13: RetinaGallery.com, James L. Perron, CRA
Figure 14: RetinaGallery.com
Figure 15: RetinaGallery.com
Figure 16: RetinaGallery.com
Figure 17: EyeRounds.org
Figure 18: Bausch and Lomb
Figure 19: Alcon Laboratories
Figure 20: Marianas Eye Institute
Figure 21: National Eye Institute, National Institutes of Health
Figure 22: National Eye Institute, National Institutes of Health
Figure 23: Welch Allyn
Figure 24: National Eye Institute, National Institutes of Health
Figure 25: Marianas Eye Institute
Figure 26: Marianas Eye Institute
Figure 27: Marianas Eye Institute
Figure 28: Zeiss
Figure 29: Zeiss

Figure 30: Marianas Eye Institute
Figure 31: Marianas Eye Institute
Figure 32: Marianas Eye Institute
Figure 33: Marianas Eye Institute
Figure 34: National Eye Institute, National Institutes of Health

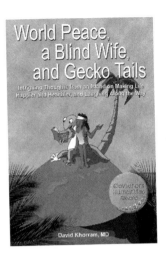

Made in the USA
Columbia, SC
17 November 2020

24764819R00111